Shoulder Surgery: Advances in Operative Techniques

Shoulder Surgery: Advances in Operative Techniques

Editor: Jennifer Ward

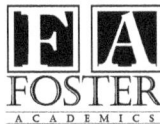

FA FOSTER
ACADEMICS

www.fosteracademics.com

www.fosteracademics.com

FA FOSTER
ACADEMICS

Cataloging-in-Publication Data

Shoulder surgery : advances in operative techniques / edited by Jennifer Ward.
    p. cm.
Includes bibliographical references and index.
ISBN 978-1-63242-757-1
1. Shoulder--Surgery. 2. Shoulder--Surgery--Techniques.
3. Surgery, Operative--Techniques. I. Ward, Jennifer.
RD557.5 .S46 2019
617.572--dc23

Foster Academics,
118-35 Queens Blvd., Suite 400,
Forest Hills, NY 11375, USA

ISBN 978-1-63242-757-1 (Hardback)

Contents

Preface

It is often said that books are a boon to mankind. They document every progress and pass on the knowledge from one generation to the other. They play a crucial role in our lives. Thus I was both excited and nervous while editing this book. I was pleased by the thought of being able to make a mark but I was also nervous to do it right because the future of students depends upon it. Hence, I took a few months to research further into the discipline, revise my knowledge and also explore some more aspects. Post this process, I begun with the editing of this book.

Shoulder surgery is a type of surgery concerned with the treatment of injured shoulders. It is most commonly used in repairing the tissues, muscles and damaged joints. Two of the major conditions in which a shoulder surgery is performed are dislocated shoulder and separated shoulder. Arthroscopic surgery and Laterjet surgery are common treatment methods used for treating a dislocated shoulder. Arthroscopic surgery is not much effective in the cases, where the shoulder bones begin to wear down even after the surgery. In such cases, a Laterjet surgery is performed. Weaver-Dunn procedure is a method for treating a separated shoulder. This book includes some of the vital pieces of work being conducted across the world, on various topics related to shoulder surgery. The various advancements in shoulder surgery are glanced at and their applications as well as ramifications are looked at in detail. Students, doctors, experts and all associated with shoulder surgery will benefit alike from this book.

I thank my publisher with all my heart for considering me worthy of this unparalleled opportunity and for showing unwavering faith in my skills. I would also like to thank the editorial team who worked closely with me at every step and contributed immensely towards the successful completion of this book. Last but not the least, I wish to thank my friends and colleagues for their support.

Editor

Superior Capsule Reconstruction: Review of a Novel Operative Technique for Management of Irreparable Rotator Cuff Tears

Alexander Golant, Daiji Kano, Tony Quach, Kevin Jiang and Jeffrey E. Rosen

Abstract

Rotator cuff tear is a common yet functionally debilitating shoulder condition. Risk factors for failure of repair or inability to repair include advancing age of the patient, chronicity of the tear, and larger tear size. Current operative management options for tears that are considered irreparable include debridement, partial repair, biceps tenotomy, interpositional grafting, tendon transfers, and reverse shoulder arthroplasty. Recently, superior capsular reconstruction has been introduced as an alternative surgical option for these tears and has demonstrated favorable short-term outcomes. However, the literature lacks studies with large numbers of patients, consistency of results, and long-term outcomes. This article reviews the anatomy and function of the rotator cuff and shoulder capsule; patho-etiology of rotator cuff tears, particularly the irreparable ones; and rationale, techniques, outcomes, and future direction of superior capsular reconstruction in the context of this clinical indication.

Keywords: shoulder, rotator cuff tear, massive rotator cuff tear, irreparable rotator cuff tear, rotator cuff repair, rotator cuff reconstruction, superior capsule reconstruction, superior capsular reconstruction

1. Introduction

Rotator cuff tears affect millions worldwide; given their age-dependent increase in prevalence, they pose a significant healthcare burden on today's aging population [1]. Chronic large to massive rotator cuff tears are often considered "irreparable" secondary to poor tissue quality, tendon retraction, and muscle atrophy and fatty infiltration [2]. Surgical options for treatment of these tears have not demonstrated consistently good outcomes [2–4]. These include attempts at relieving pain by way of debridement with or without biceps tenotomy; balancing the anterior/posterior force couples by way of partial repair; restoring cuff integrity by way of interpositional grafting; and tendon transfers. Reverse shoulder arthroplasty has been gaining popularity and demonstrates good outcomes as a treatment option for patients with rotator cuff arthropathy, but is typically reserved for the elderly patients. Massive and irreparable rotator cuff tears in younger and more active individuals, especially without significant arthritic changes of the glenohumeral joint, remain a clinical conundrum.

Recently, a new surgical procedure called superior capsular reconstruction (SCR) was described by Mihata et al., who reported promising short-term clinical outcomes in 24 shoulders (23 consecutive patients) with symptomatic irreparable rotator cuff tears [2]. Although the procedure has a strong appeal for physicians treating patients with this difficult problem and has been quickly gaining popularity, caution regarding widespread use is warranted, as large-scale and long-term data is still lacking. This chapter reviews the anatomy and function of the rotator cuff and shoulder capsule; patho-etiology of rotator cuff tears; and rationale, techniques, outcomes, and future direction of superior capsule reconstruction for irreparable tears.

2. Anatomy, biomechanics, and functions of the rotator cuff

2.1. Structural anatomy

2.1.1. Rotator cuff, interval, crescent, and cable

The rotator cuff is composed of the musculotendinous units that bound the glenohumeral joint. Its components are supraspinatus (SS), infraspinatus (IS), teres minor (TM), and subscapularis (SSC) muscles [5, 6] (**Figure 1**). The supraspinatus, which is most commonly involved in rotator cuff tears, originates on the superior aspect of the scapular body, in the supraspinous fossa, and inserts onto the anterior-superior aspect of the greater tuberosity of the humerus. The infraspinatus originates on the posterior scapular body, from the infraspinous fossa, and inserts on the posterior-superior aspect of the greater tuberosity. The teres minor, which is rarely involved in rotator cuff tears, originates from the lateral lower-half of the scapular body, inferior to the infraspinatus, and inserts on the posterior – inferior aspect of the great tuberosity and humeral head. The subscapularis, which is the largest muscle of the rotator cuff group, originates from the anterior scapular body (the subscapular fossa), runs deep to the coracoid process, and inserts onto the lesser tuberosity of the humerus. Innervation to the rotator cuff comes from the C5-6 nerve roots, with the suprascapular nerve supplying the supraspinatus and infraspinatus, axillary nerve supplying teres minor, and the upper and lower subscapular nerves supplying the subscapularis. The close interplay and confluence of the different parts of the rotator cuff creates several structures important for glenohumeral joint stability and function. These include the rotator interval, crescent, and cable.

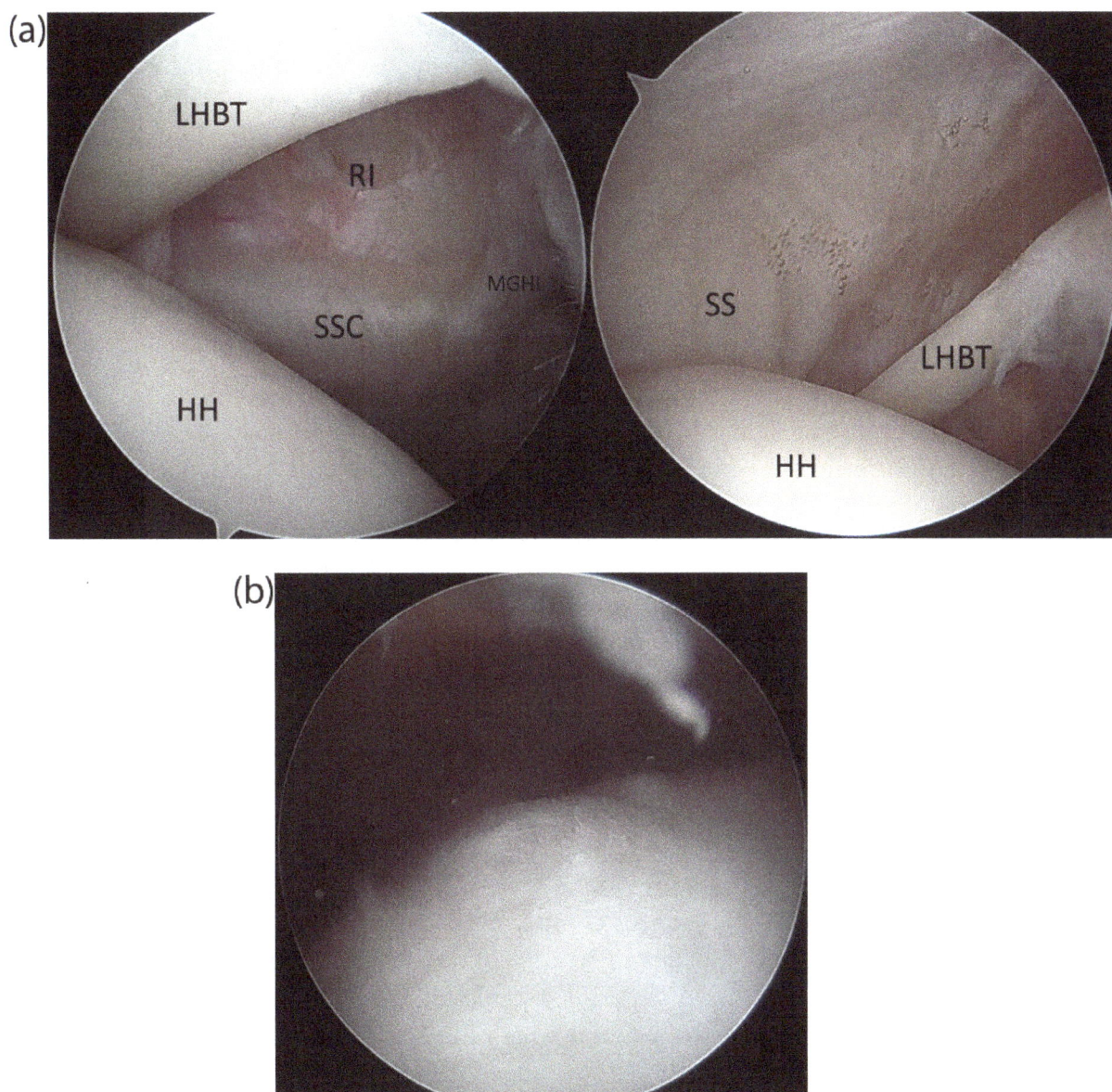

Figure 1. Arthroscopic views of the rotator cuff tendons (left shoulder). (A) Intraarticular view from the posterior portal, showing the humeral head (HH), supraspinatus (SS), subscapularis (SSC), the long-head of the biceps tendon (LHBT), the middle glenohumeral ligament (MGHL), and rotator interval (RI). (B) Bursal view of the superior rotator cuff (SS and IS)..

The rotator interval (**Figure 1A**) is the anterior triangular space between the anterior border of the supraspinatus and superior border of the subscapularis, and contains the anterior gleno-humeral joint capsule, the coracohumeral ligament (CHL), and the superior glenohumeral ligament (SGHL). The interval helps maintain the biceps tendon within the bicipital groove, and also contributes to stability of the glenohumeral joint [7, 8]. The rotator interval is also often implicated in the adhesions and contractures that occur in adhesive capsulitis of the shoulder.

The rotator crescent is a thin sheet of rotator cuff tendon, comprising the distal portions of the SS and IS insertions. The crescent is proximally bound by a thick bundle of fibers—the rotator cable—that runs perpendicular to the SS and IS fibers. Burkhart et al. described a biomechanical model of rotator cuff tears using 20 cadaver shoulders, where the rotator cable acts as a stress shield for the crescent, and the two structures form a "suspension bridge." According to this model, tears in the crescent have minimal effects on shoulder function, while those that involve the cable impair its ability to distribute the load and tension between the anterior and posterior rotator cuff and therefore its role as a dynamic stabilizer of the humeral head [9]. This concept has clinical implications as it helps guide decision making in identifying tears that can be managed non-operatively, versus those that require surgical fixation.

2.1.2. Shoulder capsule

While the rotator cuff is the main dynamic stabilizer of the glenohumeral joint, the glenohumeral joint capsule acts as a static stabilizer. It is a thin membranous structure located deep to the rotator cuff; it originates medially from the glenoid neck and inserts laterally to the anatomical neck of humerus.

The capsule is thicker anteriorly than posteriorly. The anterior capsule contains focal thickened bundles, which are called superior, middle, and anterior-inferior glenohumeral ligaments (GHL). The posterior capsule has an inferior thickening called the posterior-inferior GHL, but does not have separate ligaments further superiorly. Directly inferiorly, between the anterior-inferior and posterior-inferior glenohumeral ligaments, the capsule forms the axillary pouch, which tightens in abduction, and relaxes in adduction [3–5, 10]. Contracture and loss of normal axillary pouch volume is frequently seen in adhesive capsulitis, whereas a patulous capsule with an enlarged pouch is often seen in multi-directional shoulder instability.

The superior capsule is thin and was previously less well-studied. It originates from the glenoid neck along with its anterior-posterior counterparts, courses directly underneath the SS and anterior part of the IS, and attaches to 30–61% of surface area of the greater tuberosity (GT) [5, 10]. Nimura et al. measured superior capsule attachments in cadaveric shoulders. They reported thicker footprint at the anterior edge of SS and posterior edge of IS (5.6 ± 1.6 mm and 9.1 ± 1.7 mm, respectively), whereas the attachment was thinner at the middle area of the rotator cuff, near the posterior margin of SS (4.4 ± 1.2 mm). The authors concluded that the thinnest point of the capsule could contribute to the etiology of the initiation of degenerative rotator cuff tears [5]. The superior capsule is closely associated with the SS and IS, and typically tears together with complete tears of these tendons [1–4].

2.2. Function

The muscles of the rotator cuff help initiate movement of the shoulder joint, and also serve as the main dynamic stabilizer of this joint. Supraspinatus aids in abduction of the humerus, particularly in the scapular plane; external rotation is provided by infraspinatus (more active in adduction), and teres minor (more active in abduction); and internal rotation is the function of subscapularis. Furthermore, SS prevents abnormal inferior-superior translation of the humeral head, particularly during active arm elevation, by compressing the head into the glenoid fossa. The balancing forces between SSC anteriorly and IS and TM posteriorly provide stability in the sagittal plane, and the upward force of the deltoid is balanced by that of IS, TM, and SSC in the coronal plane [11, 12].

The shoulder capsule provides static stability, serving to prevent excessive translation of the humeral head relative to the glenoid [5, 10]. The anterior capsule prevents anterior translation, while the posterior prevents posterior translation. The function of the superior capsule was previously poorly understood and continues to be studied. Ishihara et al. demonstrated in a biomechanical study that the superior capsule plays an important role in passive stability in all directions, and cutting it significantly increases abnormal translation, especially superiorly [10]. This can lead to a decrease in the acromiohumeral distance—a finding commonly seen in patients with chronic massive superior cuff tears as well as cuff-tear arthropathy [2] (**Figure 2**).

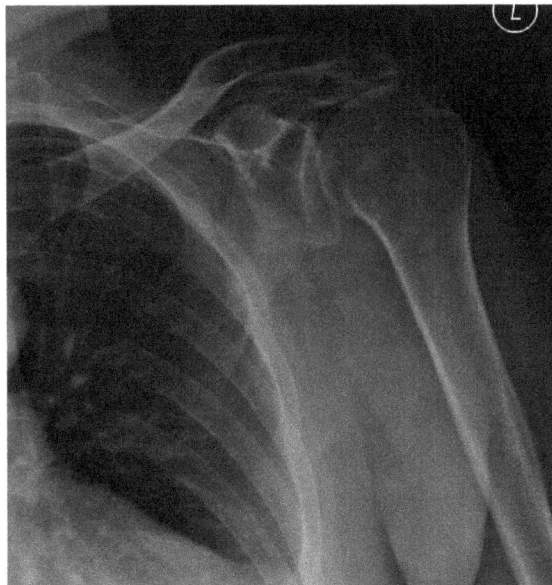

Figure 2. Anterior-posterior plain radiograph of a left shoulder with rotator cuff arthropathy. Note the "high-riding" humeral head, with a decreased acromiohumeral distance, and interrupted Shenton's line at the inferior aspect of the glenohumeral joint.

3. Etiology of rotator cuff tears

While a significant number of rotator cuff tear cases present to the physician after a traumatic episode, most tears do not occur in a setting of a normal tendon. Preexisting degenerative changes are usually found in the torn tendons, and the injury that leads to clinical presentation is likely the "straw that breaks the camel's back." A number of both intrinsic and extrinsic pathways and risk factors are thought to contribute to chronic degeneration and weakening of the cuff tendons, as described below (**Table 1**).

The main intrinsic mechanism pathway is thought to be tenocyte apoptosis and inflammation resulting from chronic microtrauma to the rotator cuff tendons. Advancing age is the most common reason for this mechanism, and age has been found to be the strongest risk factor for rotator cuff disease. This is thought to be due to the combination of age-related degenerative changes and accumulation of microtrauma and macrotrauma over the course of an individual's lifetime [3, 4]. Older patients are also more likely to develop larger tears; Gumina et al.

Strong association	Controversial or weak association
Age (particularly >60)	Peripartum Hormonal changes
Smoking (dose and time-dependent)	Dominant side
Family history	Postural abnormalities
Previous history of tear	
Trauma	
Hypercholesterolemia	
Heavy labor and overhead athletes (chronic wear-and-tear)	

Table 1. Risk factors for rotator cuff pathology.

reported a mean age of 59 years in a group of 586 patients undergoing arthroscopic tear repair, with those older than 60 being twice as likely to develop large and massive tears [13].

Tendon degeneration and poor healing potential are exacerbated by hypovascularity, which is worsened not only with advancing age, but also with smoking, and certain other conditions [4]. Smoking has a strong dose and time-dependent association with both the prevalence and size of tears; it negatively affects the vascularity of tendons, thereby predisposing them to tears and preventing healing [3, 4]. Similarly, hypercholesterolemia has been implicated in rotator cuff disease. The mechanism here is thought to be deposition of cholesterol by-products within the rotator cuff tendons, leading to worsening of biomechanical properties of the tendon and increasing the risk of tearing [14].

Genetic predisposition may also play a role. Patients diagnosed relatively early in life (before age 40) often have a family history of rotator cuff disease [3]. Particularly in irreparable tears, studies have shown expression of genes that favor fatty atrophy and fibrosis and inhibit myogenesis [15].

The most commonly accepted extrinsic mechanism for rotator cuff disease was originally described by Neer in his classic article from 1972, *Anterior Acromioplasty for the Chronic Impingement Syndrome in the Shoulder: a Preliminary Report*, and has guided clinical approach to management of impingement and rotator cuff tears ever since, although validity of some of these concepts has been challenged in the recent years. Neer suggested that repetitive contact between the rotator cuff tendons and the underside of the coracoacromial arch (which includes the anterolateral acromion, coracoacromial ligament, and the coracoid) results in trauma to the tendon, which produces the clinical entities of subacromial or subcoracoid impingement, and, in its more advanced stages, tendon tears [16]. Acromial morphology (hooked versus flat) and presence of subacromial enthesophytes have also been proposed to be contributing factors to symptomatic cuff disease, and surgical approach directed at increasing the space under coracoacromial arch by way of acromioplasty and coracoacromial ligament release has been advocated [17]. However, recent studies have questioned the benefit of these procedures [18], and attention has been directed to position and dynamic function of the scapula, as a contributor to rotator cuff impingement and tears [19]. Therefore, postural abnormalities and peri-scapular muscle strength have received greater recent attention as potentially contributing risk factor that can and should be addressed in management of rotator cuff disease.

4. Outcomes of rotator cuff repair

Rotator cuff repair was originally performed with open, and subsequently mini-open, techniques, which have produces good results, including restoration of shoulder strength and function. Advent and popularization of arthroscopy have allowed for a less invasive method of rotator cuff repair, contributing to decreased postoperative pain and more rapid return of motion. Other modern advancements, such as improved instrumentation, as well as stronger and more biocompatible suture and anchor materials, have led to new surgical techniques, such as a double-row rotator repair, which may contribute to better healing and possibly improved outcomes, especially for larger tears. Multiple clinical studies of arthroscopic repair have shown good to excellent results in as many as 90% of patients postoperatively, even including those with large and massive tears [20–23]. A recent systemic review and meta-analysis by McElvany et al. [24] included 108 clinical studies and showed postoperative clinical outcomes scores improved by an average of 103% of the preoperative scores. However, despite the overall good results, this same study found that 26.6% of the repairs failed to heal. Failure to heal may not (and often does not) affect short-term results, but may lead to deterioration of shoulder function after 2 years post-repair. Risk factors for failure of the rotator cuff tear to heal after surgery include preoperative fatty infiltration of the muscle, older age, and increased tear size. As many as 50% of larger (≥3 cm) tears may fail to heal after repair.

One of the most important predictors for failure of rotator cuff repair, along with tear size, is muscle atrophy and fatty infiltration (**Figure 3**). Most common system used to classify fatty degeneration of rotator cuff muscles was described by Goutallier et al. [25]. Even small and medium tears are at risk for failure after repair with as little as grade 2 muscle degeneration [26]. Shoulders with more severe (grade 3 or 4) degeneration, where more than 50% of muscle volume is replaced by fat, are at a very high risk of poor outcomes, since, even if tendon repair and healing to bone is achieved, dynamic function of the rotator cuff muscle-tendon unit remains compromised.

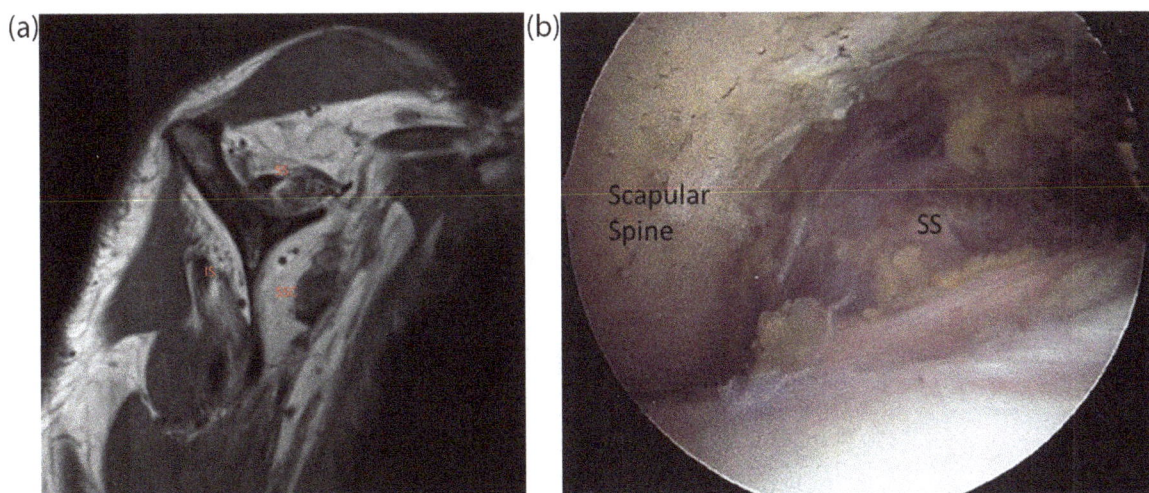

Figure 3. Fatty atrophy of the superior rotator cuff. (A) Sagittal MRI view of a right shoulder showing severe fatty degeneration (more than 50% of muscle volume replaced by fat) of the supraspinatus (SS), infraspinatus (IS), and subscapularis (SSC) muscles. (B) Arthroscopic view of the supraspinatus (SS), demonstrating severe muscle atrophy (view from a posterolateral subacromial portal in the right shoulder).

Therefore, due to poor healing potential and low likelihood of restoration of good cuff function, chronic large (3–5 cm) and massive (>5 cm) tears, especially those with Goutallier 2 or greater atrophy, may be considered irreparable. Other types of tears that are considered irreparable include tears with significant retraction of the tendon (medial to the glenoid), poor tendon quality for repair, and poor bone quality at the greater tuberosity attachment site (**Figure 4**). Attempts at repair of tears with these features should be approached with guarded expectations.

Those rotator cuff tears that fail to heal or are irreparable frequently go on to a clinical condition called cuff tear arthropathy (CTA) (**Figure 2**). This is a specific form of shoulder arthritis resulting from rotator cuff deficiency. Due to the failure and absence of superior restraint, the humeral head typically migrates superiorly, and eventually articulates with the acromion. Over time this leads to wear of the acromion, destruction of the humeral head cartilage, and eventually the glenoid cartilage as well. Patients typically present with significant pain, weakness, and crepitus with range of motion, and sometimes even pseudoparalysis—severe inability to elevate the shoulder. Once advanced CTA develops, the only surgical solution available to treat it (other than fusion of the shoulder joint) is a reverse total shoulder replacement (**Figure 5**).

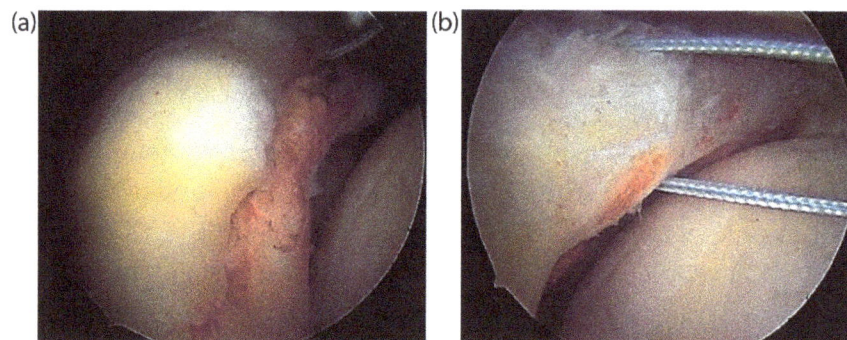

Figure 4. Massive tear of the superior rotator cuff, not amenable to repair. (A) Note poor tissue quality of the tendon stump, and retraction medial to the glenoid rim. (B) Despite extensive releases, this tendon stump could not be mobilized even to the medial margin of the greater tuberosity.

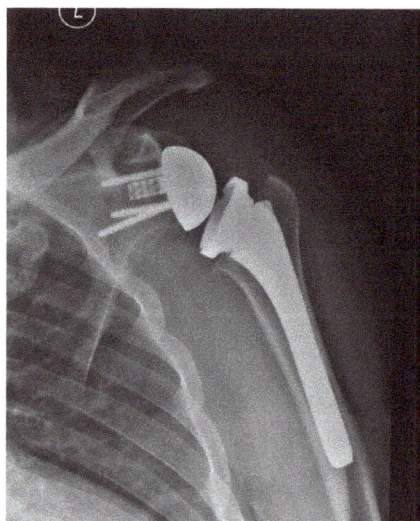

Figure 5. Reverse shoulder replacement in a 60 year-old man, performed for symptomatic advanced cuff-tear arthropathy.

5. Treatment options for irreparable rotator cuff tears

The treatment of massive and irreparable rotator cuff tears is challenging. Surgical options include partial repair with marginal convergence, debridement with biceps tenotomy, graft interposition, tendon transfer, reverse total shoulder, and now superior capsular reconstruction. Partial repair of the inferior half of the infraspinatus was originally described by Burkhart et al. in 1994, with the goal restoring a balanced anterior-posterior force couple in the shoulder [27]. Multiple studies which analyzed surgery for massive cuff tears with combinations of partial repair, marginal convergence, debridement, and biceps tenotomy have shown mixed results, typically with good outcomes early on, but persistent strength deficit in elevation, and deterioration of clinical results over time. For example, Shon et al. performed partial repair and marginal convergence techniques in 31 patients and found initial improvement in clinical outcome scores, whereas 2-year follow-up showed a dissatisfaction rate of 50% [28]. Fatty infiltration of the infraspinatus was found to be a negative predictor of outcome in these patients.

Graft interposition techniques to bridge irreparable rotator cuff defects have been described using autograft, allograft, xenograft, and synthetic materials. A systematic review of these techniques found a lack of high quality comparative studies. The limited studies available show improvement in clinical outcomes in all graft types [29], with allograft, xenograft, and synthetic grafts having the appeal of no harvest site morbidity, compared to autograft. On the other hand, significant inflammatory reactions have been reported with the use of xenografts as well as allografts [30], and therefore caution must be used. Just as with other surgeries for massive cuff tear, significant fatty atrophy leads to significantly lower healing rates after graft interposition repairs. Finally, interpositional grafts may need to be placed through an open approach, which runs the increased disk of damage to the deltoid muscle, potentially making subsequent revision surgery more difficult and less successful. In summary, due to lack of high quality comparative studies on the use of graft interposition for cuff repair, the potential benefits of this procedure must be weighed against the cost, risks, and potential future complications of this approach.

Several tendon transfer procedures have been described for the treatment of massive irreparable rotator cuff tears. Tendon transfers are typically performed in younger patients without glenohumeral arthritis and good range of motion. The most common transfers used for posterosuperior tears are latissimus dorsi and lower trapezius transfers. Clinical studies show latissimus dorsi transfer provides significant pain relief after tendon transfer, whereas functional results are more unpredictable [31]. Lower trapezius transfer anatomically provides a more direct line of pull compared to latissimus dorsi transfer; however, limited clinical evidence is available to show improvement in pain and function.

Reverse total shoulder arthroplasty (RTSA) is a semiconstrained reverse ball and socket prosthesis which helps improve the biomechanical efficiency of the deltoid muscle by lengthening its lever arm. The design provides inherent glenohumeral stability and lowers the humeral head to increase deltoid tension, which allows this muscle to elevate the arm without a functional rotator cuff. While elevation is typically restored after RTSA, active rotation of the shoulder is not as easily recovered as it relies on presence of the anterior-posterior components of the cuff. Overall, clinical studies have shown significant improvements in pain, motion, and functional scores in patients treated for cuff-tear arthropathy. However, implant longevity is a concern, as are functional limitations imposed by this surgery. Due to these limitations, reverse shoulder arthroplasty is typically reserved for patients in their 60s, 70s, and older [32].

6. Rationale, indications, and contraindications for superior capsule reconstruction (SCR)

The main reason to consider superior capsule reconstruction (SCR) is as an alternative to reverse shoulder arthroplasty or tendon transfers in patients with irreparable superior rotator cuff tears, with or without early cuff tear arthropathy. In this procedure a graft tissue is attached to the superior glenoid and the greater tuberosity, thereby spanning the superior aspect of the glenohumeral joint (**Figure 6**). The biomechanical rationale behind this surgery is debated. One proposed rationale is a tenodesis effect between the glenoid and the humeral head, which helps regain the stabilizing effect to the glenohumeral articulation normally conferred by the superior capsule and the rotator cuff [2]. This has been called the "reverse trampoline" effect. The other proposed mechanism is that the inserted graft acts a spacer between the humeral head and the underside of the acromion, essentially keeping the head depressed by

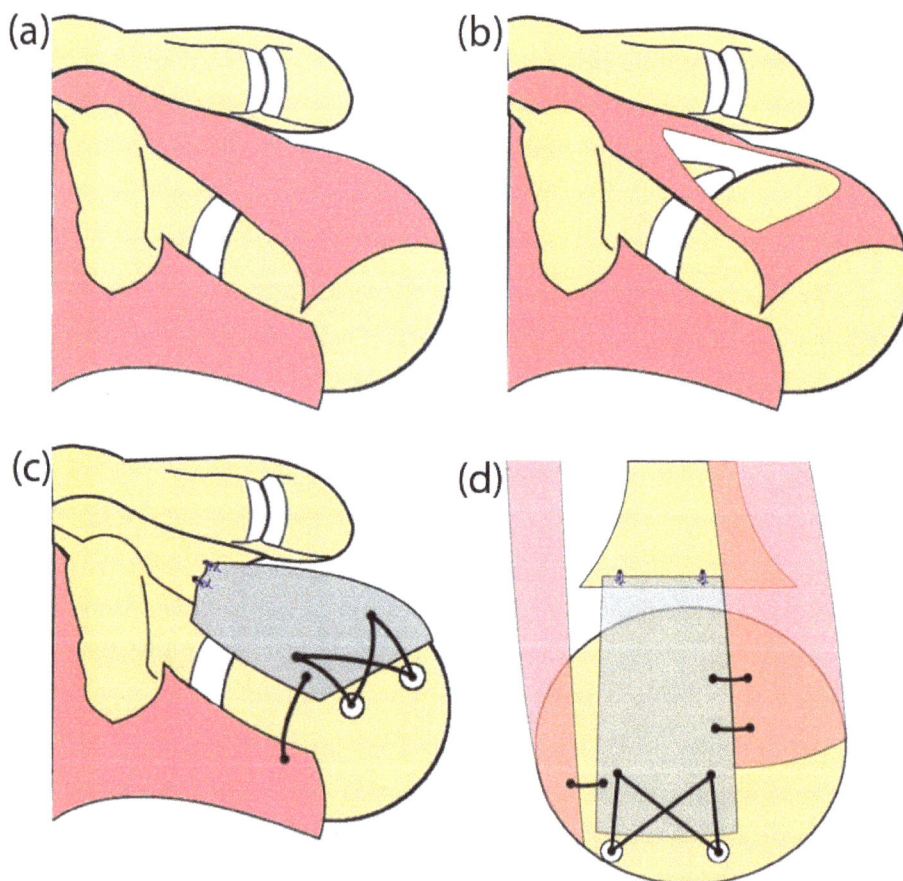

Figure 6. Schematic drawing, showing a shoulder with a normal superior rotator cuff (A), a large and irreparable defect of the superior cuff (B), and after a SCR (C and D).

way occupying the space above it. Biomechanical cadaveric studies by Mihata and colleagues have shown that SCR does restore superior translation to physiologic conditions [33]; and also that increased thickness of the graft improves stability [34]. These studies lend credence to both theories regarding biomechanical function of SCR; indeed both factors may be at play.

Indications for this surgery currently include physiologically young (absolute age has not been determined) and relatively active patients with symptomatic irreparable superior rotator cuff, with intact anterior-posterior force couples, and no or minimal glenohumeral arthritic wear. Young patients with moderate cartilage wear and symptoms primarily related to cuff function may be considered for SCR, in lieu of RTSA, but guarded expectation are warranted with more severe arthritic wear. SCR may also be an attractive option for previous failed cuff repair, in a setting of poor tissue quality, fatty infiltration, and other factors that may result in tear irreparability.

Absolute contraindications include infection, neuropathic disease of the shoulder, and neurologic disorders significantly affecting function of the deltoid muscle. Relative contraindications include advanced arthritis, tears of the anterior/posterior rotator cuff, as well as unwillingness or inability to comply with postoperative immobilization and rehabilitation protocol.

7. Technique

Arthroscopic reconstruction using tensor fascia lata was initially proposed by Mihata et al. [2]. Several other authors have reported SCR using acellular dermal allograft [35–39]. An arthroscopic technique is typically used for this procedure, but an open technique may be used in cases of difficult arthroscopic exposure or for surgeons less familiar with arthroscopic techniques. We describe our preferred technique for arthroscopic superior capsular reconstruction.

7.1. Surgical positioning

Surgery is typically performed in an ambulatory setting, under combination general and regional anesthesia. After induction of anesthesia, and prior to positioning (with the patient supine on the operating table), the shoulder should be examined for passive motion and stability. Manipulation of the shoulder to regain motion should be performed as needed. We prefer a beach-chair position with the arm supported by a hydraulic arm positioner device, but a lateral decubitus with balanced suspension-traction may also be used.

7.2. Diagnostic arthroscopy and associated procedures

Standard posterior portal is used to enter the glenohumeral joint, and an anterior portal is established in the rotator interval. A thorough diagnostic arthroscopy of the glenohumeral joint is performed, and pathologic lesions are addressed as needed. Particular attention must be paid to the integrity of the subscapularis tendon, which needs to be repaired if significantly torn. If the biceps tendon is still present in the joint (more often than not there is a chronic tear and absence of the long head), it needs to be removed from the superior glenoid, so that it does not block graft placement; a tenotomy or tenodesis is performed. Any loose bodies should be removed, and synovectomy is performed as needed. Chondroplasty may be performed for frayed and unstable cartilage flaps on the humeral head and glenoid.

The camera is then repositioned into the subacromial space. Subacromial portals are created, typically one anterolaterally and one posterolaterally. A bursectomy is performed, and the rotator cuff tear is then carefully evaluated, characterized and mobilized, ensuring that a repair is not possible or not advisable. A superior capsular reconstruction is considered if there is a massive full-thickness tear of the supraspinatus, without or without infraspinatus tear, that cannot be repaired, and the glenohumeral joint does not show severe degenerative changes (**Figure 7**).

Once a decision is made to perform a SCR, an acromioplasty should be performed, to increase working space for graft placement and fixation, and also to decrease the risk of graft tissue abrasion postoperatively [40]. Any osteophytes off the inferior aspect of the AC joint need to be resected as well (**Figure 8**). We always attempt to preserve the CA ligament, if possible, so as not to disrupt the coracoacromial arch.

We also prefer at this time to place #2 braided sutures into the upper borders of the intact cuff posteriorly (teres minor or infraspinatus) and anteriorly (subscapularis or intact anterior fibers of the supraspinatus); these are used, after graft fixation, to repair the native cuff to the patch, side to side. Additionally, if there is any significant cuff tissue remaining medially, overlying the glenoid rim, it can be tagged with a #2 suture through a Neviaser portal, and pulled up for better visualization of the superior glenoid (**Figure 9**).

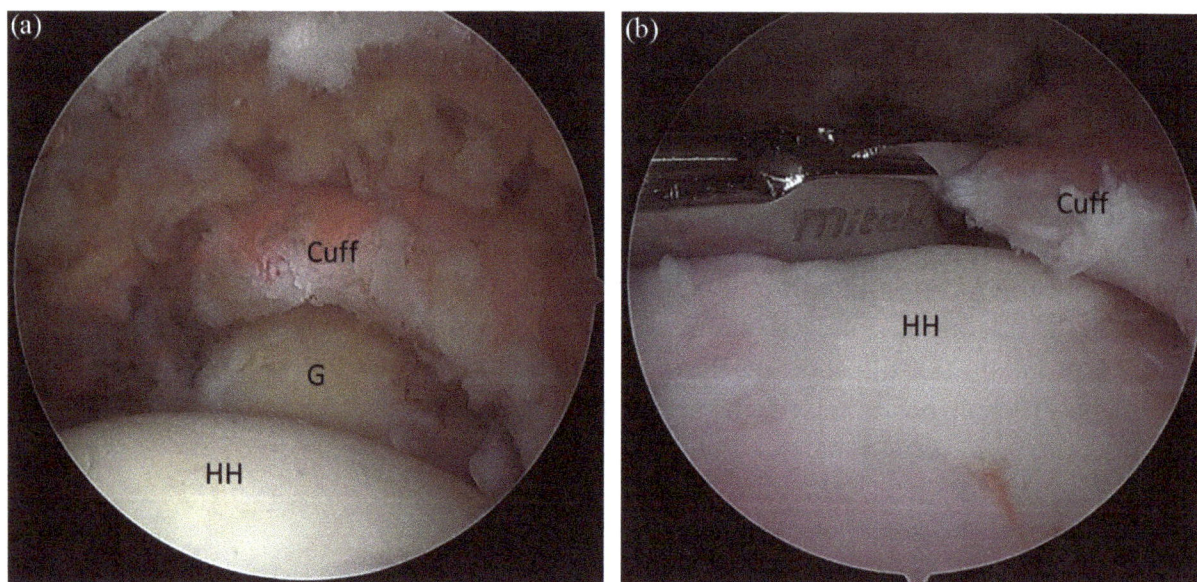

Figure 7. Massive and irreparable rotator cuff tear in the left shoulder of a 70 year old active male (view from posterolateral portal). (A) Note severely retracted massive tear of the superior cuff (SS and IS), with relatively normal articular cartilage both on the glenoid and the humeral head. (B) Even after extensive releases, the tendon stump is not adequately mobile for primary repair (HH—humeral head; G—glenoid).

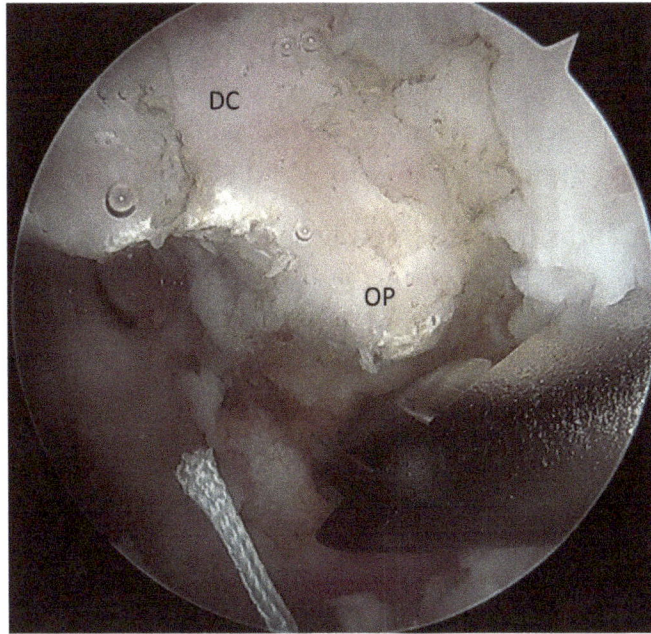

Figure 8. An inferior osteophyte (OP) is being resected off the distal clavicle (DC), to avoid impingement and abrasion of the graft postoperatively.

7.3. Bony preparation, anchor placements

Any residual soft tissue on the superior glenoid neck and greater tuberosity is removed using a motorized shaver and/or electrocautery wand. To maximize healing potential, the superior glenoid neck and greater tuberosity are burred down to bleeding bone.

Medial anchors are placed on the superior glenoid, approximately 2–4 mm medial to the rim, taking care to ensure good bone purchase and avoid intraarticular penetration. Anchors are placed as far anterior and posterior as possible to provide adequate spread and coverage for

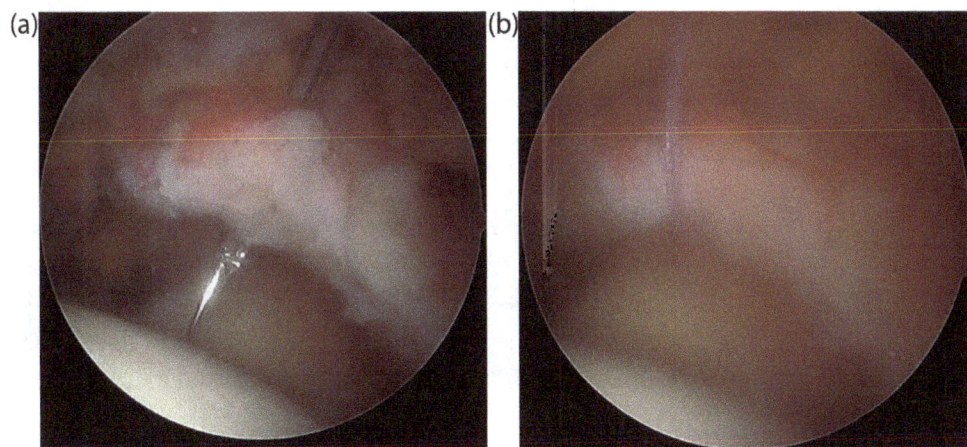

Figure 9. (A) A penetrating suture passer is inserted through the Neviaser portal and is used to pass a tagging suture through the rotator cuff tendon stump. (B) The rotator cuff can then be pulled up, to allow better visualization of and instrumentation on the glenoid neck.

the medial graft fixation on the glenoid. Typically two anchors, each double loaded with a #2 braided suture, are placed, in the region between the 10 and 2 o'clock positions (**Figure 10A** and **B**), but a third anchor may need to be added for very large defects (**Figure 10C**). Appropriate trajectory for anchor placement should be confirmed prior to drilling, and can typically be achieved from the anterior, posterior and Neviaser portals.

On the humeral head, graft fixation is accomplished using a double row transosseous equivalent technique. Prior to graft passage, medial row greater tuberosity anchors placed, just lateral to the articular margin (**Figure 11**). We prefer to use anchors preloaded with #2 suture-tape, non-sliding. As on the glenoid, two anchors are typically used, but a third one may be needed in large shoulders with large defects.

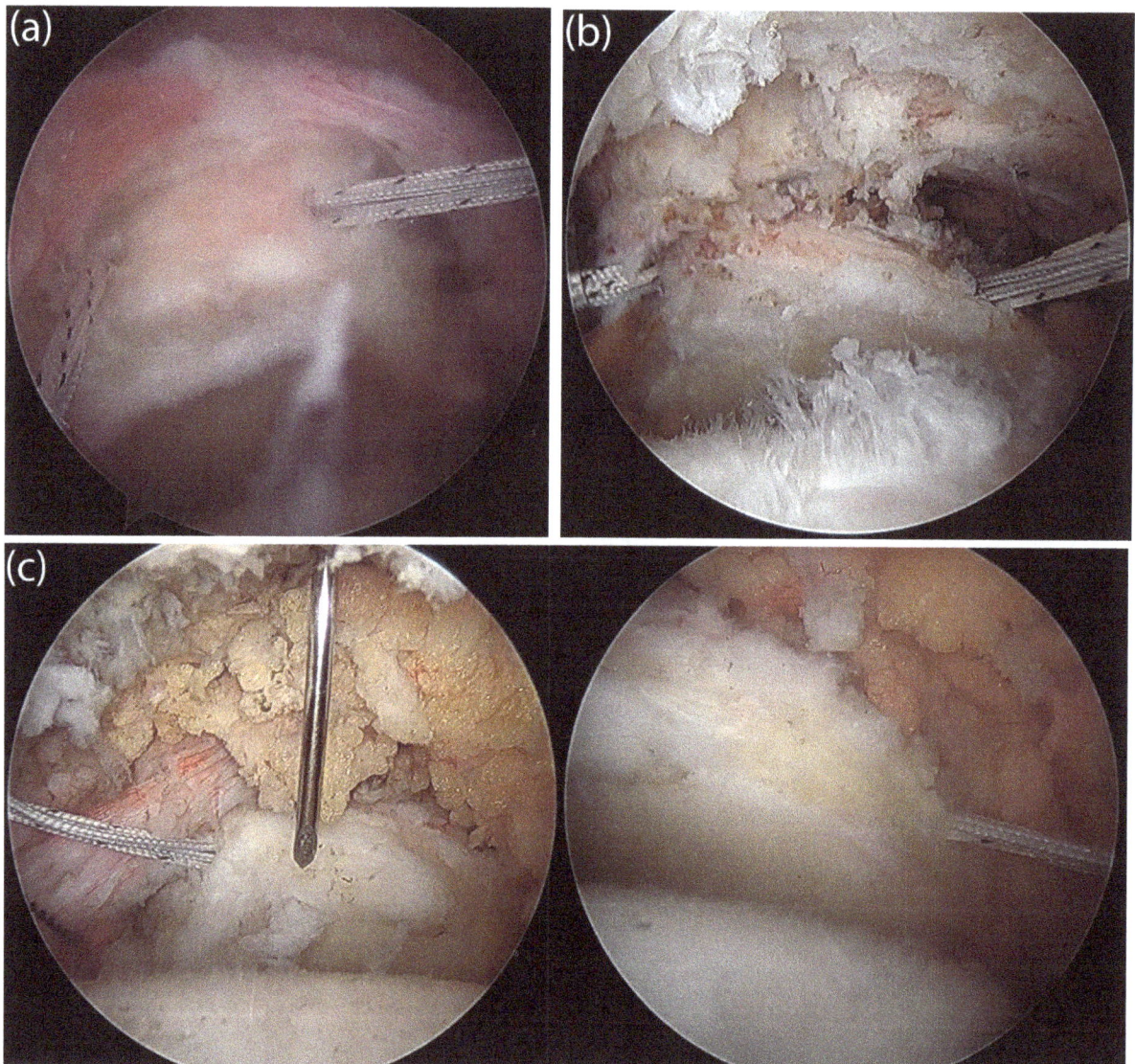

Figure 10. Glenoid anchors. Each one is double-loaded with a #2 braided suture. Note the anchor position approximately 2–4 mm medial to the rim, and the trajectory of insertion (away from the articular cartilage). The spread between the anchors can be narrow (A) for smaller defects, or wide (B) for larger ones. Sometimes three anchors may need to be placed (C), for massive tears involving both the SS and IS. In this case, a Neviaser portal helps with proper trajectory for the middle anchor, as shown by the spinal needle.

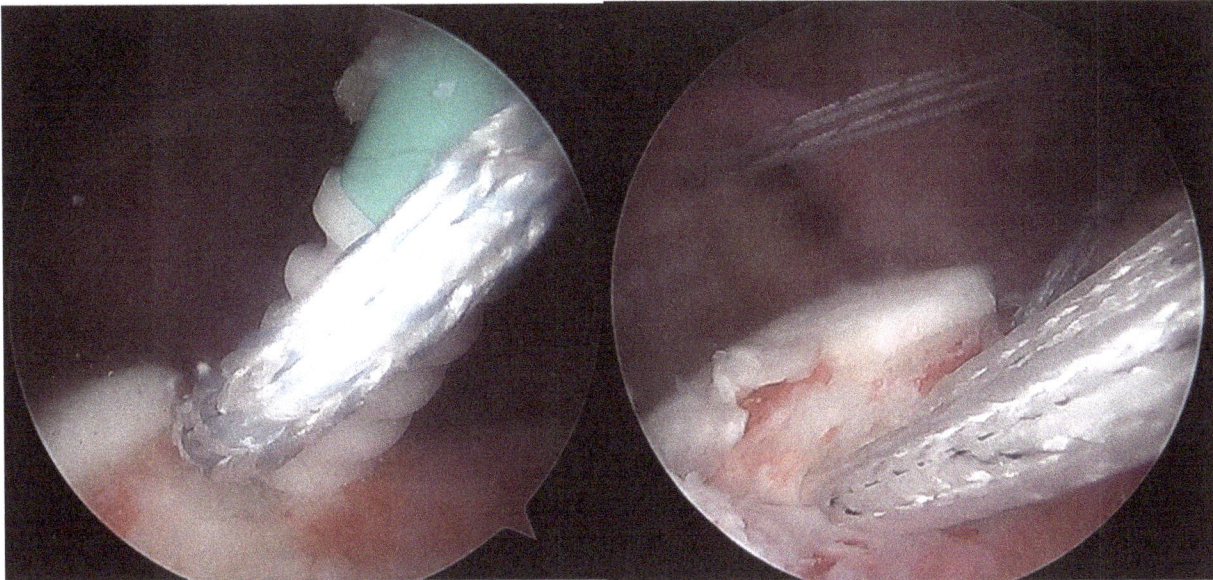

Figure 11. Medial row greater tuberosity (GT) anchors are inserted. The anterior anchor is placed just posterior to the bicipital groove, and the posterior anchor is at the posterior-most extent of the exposed tuberosity. Both are pre-loaded with a suture-tape, and placed adjacent to the articular margin of the humeral head. Note how the surface of the GT has been decorticated down to bleeding bone.

7.4. Graft sizing and preparation

Once all the anchors are placed, distances between them are measured. First the anterior-posterior distance is measured for the glenoid anchors and tuberosity anchors. Then the medial-lateral distance is measured between the glenoid and tuberosity anchors, obtaining one measurement anteriorly, and one posteriorly. A calibrated probe is used to make these measurements (**Figure 12**). In our opinion, in order to obtain the graft size that will provide appropriate stabilizing affect without overtightening the glenohumeral articulation, the shoulder should be positioned in neutral rotation and approximately 20–30° of abduction for the measurement, and during subsequent graft fixation.

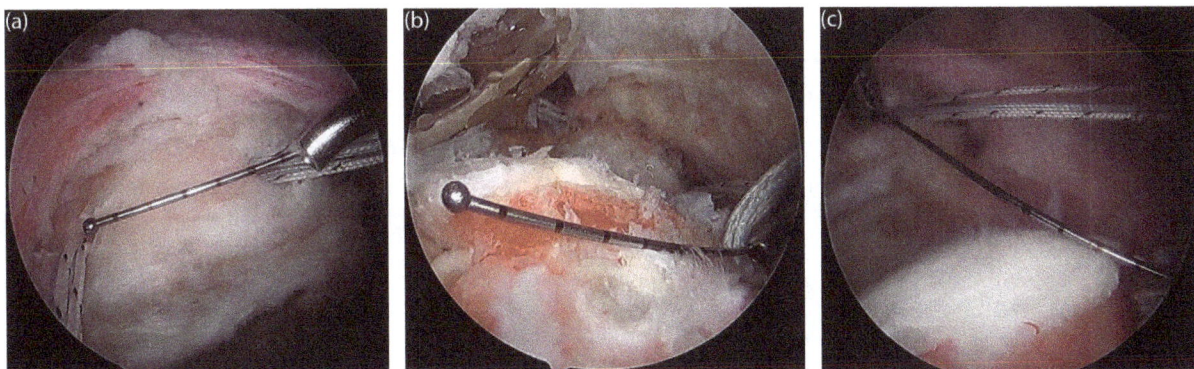

Figure 12. Measuring distances between the anchors using a calibrated probe. (A) Distance between the glenoid anchors. (B) Distance between the medial GT anchors. (C) Distance between the glenoid and GT anchors (posterior, viewing from the anterolateral portal).

Next the graft if prepared. We use an acellular human dermal graft (Arthroflex by Arthex, Inc., Naples, FL), but an autograft, such as tensior fascia lata, may also be harvested and used. Whichever graft is used, it is now sized and prepared on the back table. The graft is cut to allow a 5 mm margin medially, anteriorly and posteriorly and a 10 mm margin laterally. The dimensions of the anchor configuration are then carefully marked on the graft using a marking pen (**Figure 13**).

At this point, all the sutures must be brought out through one of the subacromial portals in preparation for graft passage. We prefer to view from the posterior or posterolateral portal, and use the anterolateral portal for graft passage. Sometimes this portal must be slightly increased in size, and a flexible cannula, which can be cut along one of its sides (such as the Arthex Passport) can be helpful.

The graft is brought close to the shoulder, carefully supported on a sterile Mayo stand. The sutures from the glenoid anchors are passed through the medial edge of the graft. Simple configuration can be used, but we prefer to place each sets of sutures in a criss-crossing mattress configuration (one vertically and one horizontally), creating a Mason-Allen type configuration. One limb from each suture set is tied to a limb from another suture set (off a different color), and the knot tails are cut. This leaves two suture limbs (one of each color) on the anterior-medial and posterior-medial edges of the graft, which, when tensioned, create a pulley effect on the graft, allowing it to be drawn into the joint (**Figures 14** and **15**).

At this time it is possible to either place the tuberosity medial row sutures through the graft, or instead place a suture loop (such as Arthrex Fiberlink) which would aide with the passage of those sutures later. The advantage of the latter approach is minimizing suture traffic in the lateral subacromial portal, and avoiding suture entanglement. We prefer this technique (**Figure 14**), and temporarily park the medial row tuberosity sutures in the anterior and posterior portals, while the graft is being passed.

7.5. Graft passage

The suture pulley system previously created on the medial side of the graft with the glenoid sutures is now tensioned. The graft may need to be partially folded to allow it to pass through the cannula, or the cannula may be removed (if it was pre-cut). Also, a blunt tissue grasper can be used to pinch the graft medially to ease the delivery and transport of the graft through the cannula. The graft is visualized entering the joint, and moving medially until it sits flush on the superior glenoid neck, covering the rim (**Figure 16A** and **B**). It may be necessary to help unfold the anterior and posterior edges of the graft once its fully inside, in case they get folded in.

7.6. Graft fixation

The sutures from the glenoid anchors are then tied arthroscopically to secure the graft to the glenoid neck. The tails of those sutures may be passed up through the remnant of the native cuff, to bring it down to the medial edge of the graft, helping create a biologic seal over this area (**Figure 16C**).

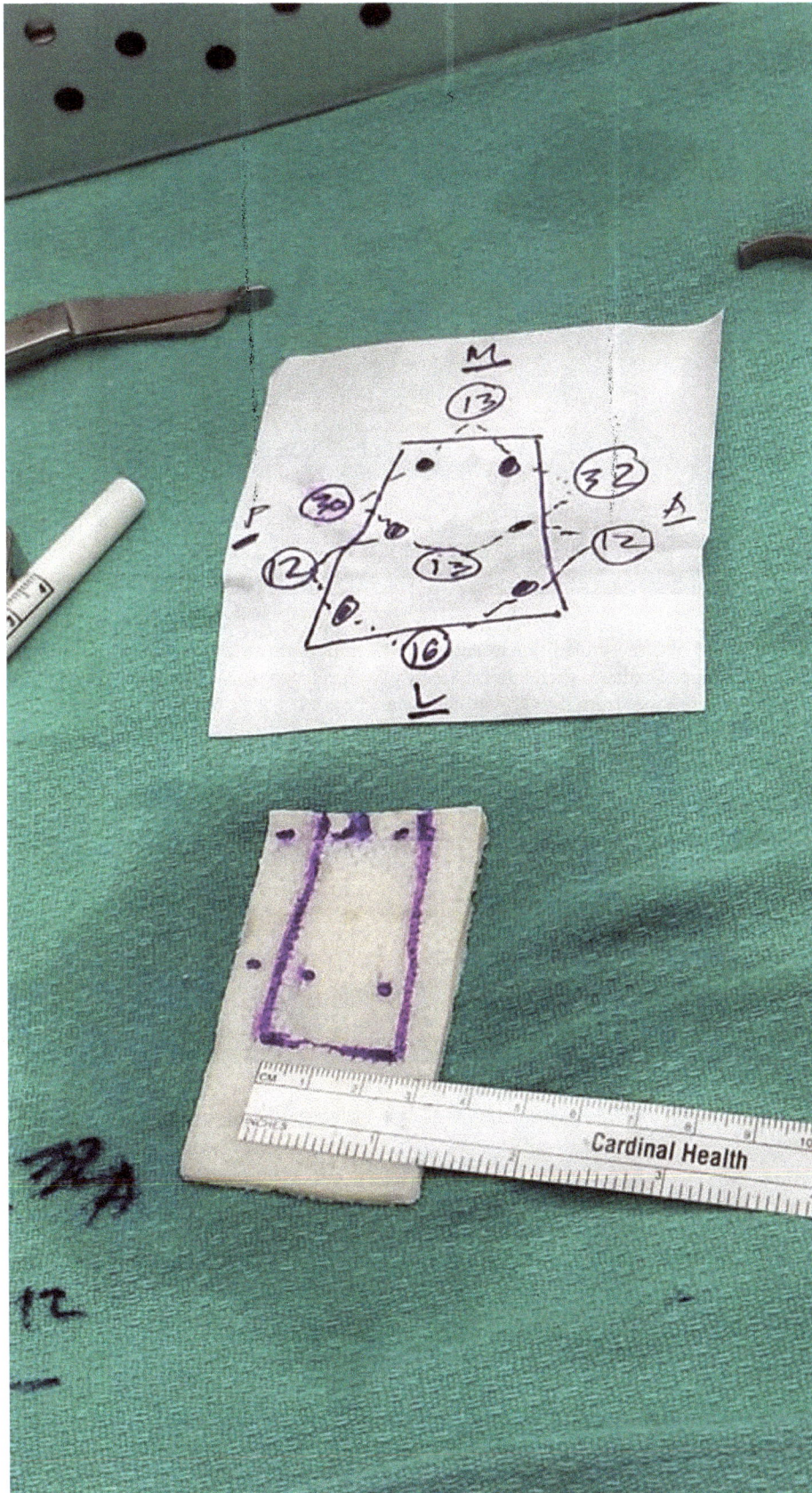

Figure 13. Graft measurement. It is important not to cut the graft too short. 5 mm extra is left on the medial, anterior, and posterior edges, whereas laterally 10 mm extra distance is left to allow coverage over the GT footprint.

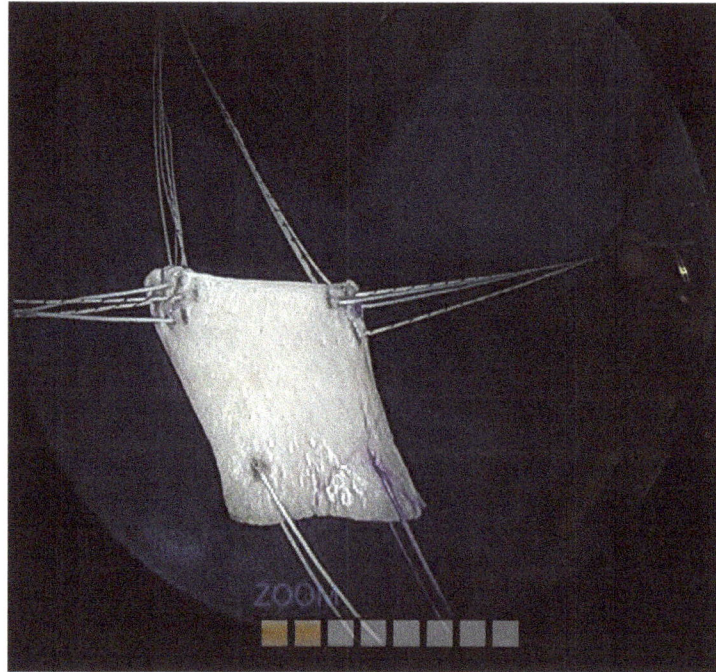

Figure 14. Suture placement into the graft prior to shuttling. Glenoid sutures are placed in a horizontal and vertical mattress configurations, perpendicular to each other. Laterally, we prefer to place a suture-loop (Arthrex Fiberlink), for subsequent shuttling of suture-tapes from the GT medial row anchors.

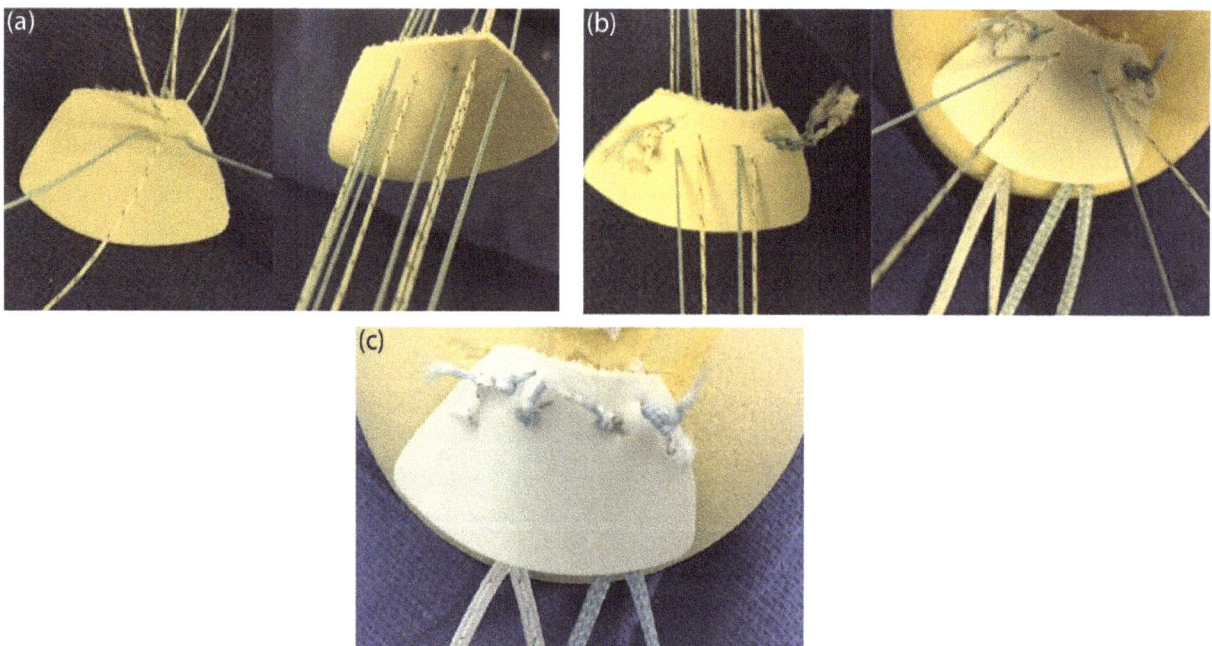

Figure 15. Model demonstration of the step-by-step process of glenoid suture placement and tying. (A) All suture limbs from each anchor are placed in a mattress configuration, perpendicular to each other. (B) One limb from each suture is tied to a limb from the other suture (different color), and this creates a double-pulley system, which helps shuttle the graft to its attachment points on the glenoid. (C) Final construct, with all glenoid sutures tied.

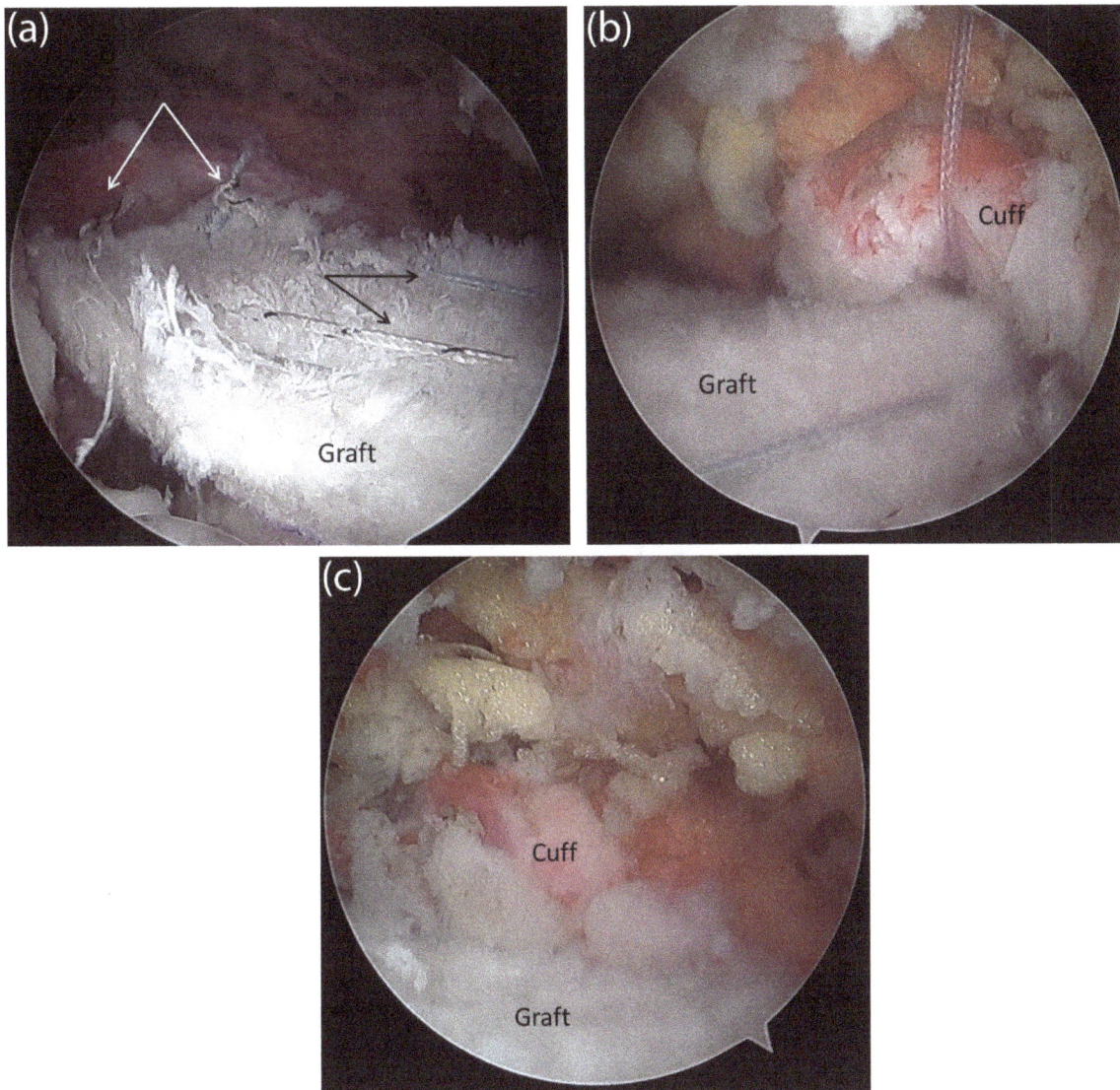

Figure 16. Arthroscopic view of graft fixation to the glenoid. (A) The graft is pulled in using the double-pulley system, which is created by tying one limb of each suture to the other one from the same anchor (white arrows); the remaining limbs act as pulley sutures (black arrows), to cinch the graft onto the superior glenoid rim. (B) Note the ability to pull up the remnant of the superior cuff, with a previously placed free suture, via the Neviaser portal, for improved visualization. (C) After the sutures from the glenoid anchors are tied, securing the graft to the glenoid, the remnant cuff tissue can be tied down to the graft, using those suture tails. This creates a nice biologic seal over the medial part of the SCR construct.

Then the tuberosity medial row sutures are passed through the graft using the previously pre-loaded suture-loop, if they haven't been already placed outside the shoulder. Both limbs of the sutures from the medial GT anchors are passed through the graft, from inferior to superior, one at the anterior and one at the posterior pre-determined spots (**Figure 17A**). Finally, these suture-tapes are brought over the lateral-most extent of the graft in a criss-cross fashion, and secured just past the lateral margin of the tuberosity with knotless anchors (**Figure 17B–D**). Prior to setting final tension and fixating the graft laterally, proper shoulder position of neutral rotation and slight abduction (20–30°) needs to be ensured.

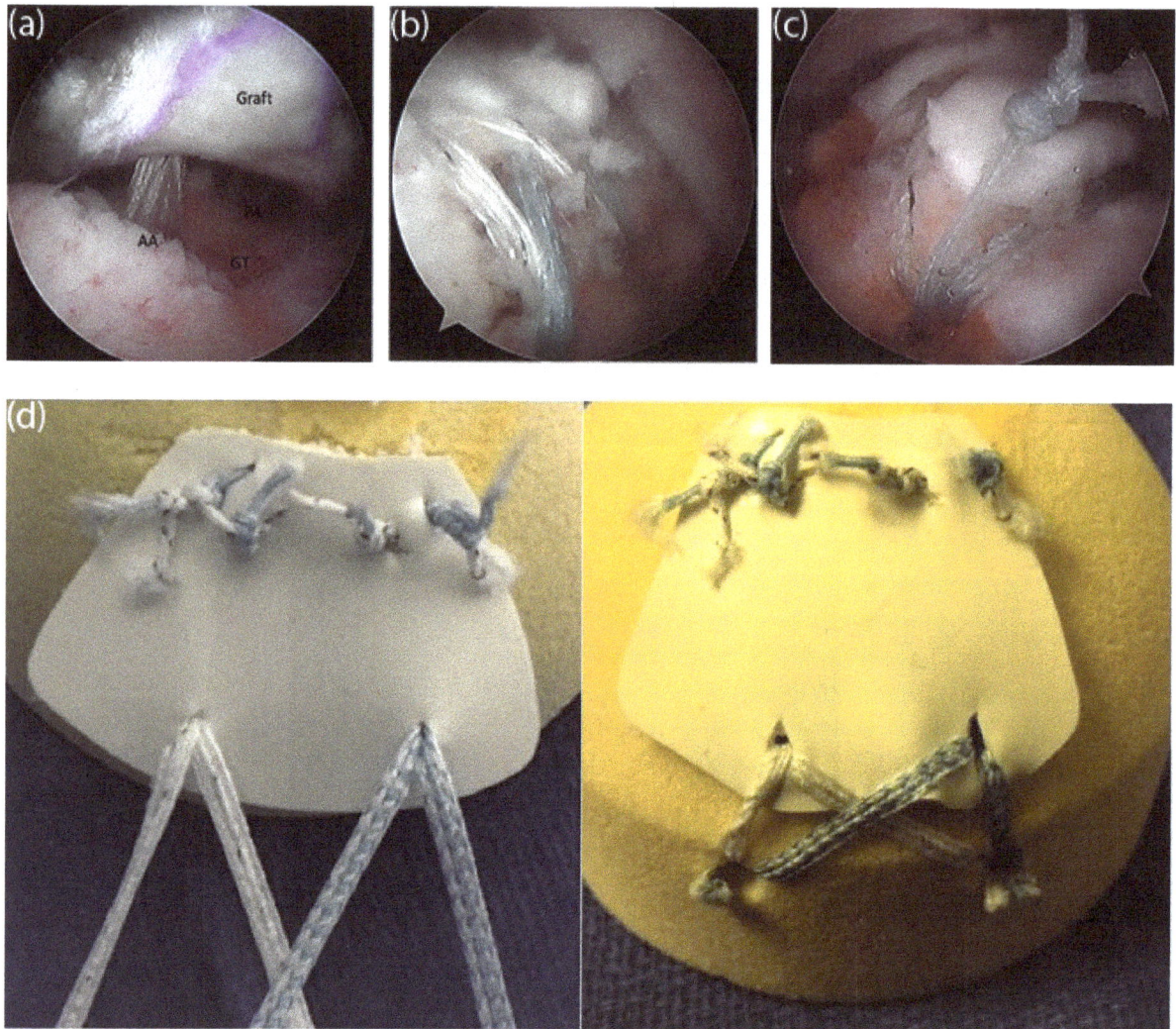

Figure 17. Graft fixation to the humeral head. (A) Suture-tapes from the medial row greater tuberosity anchors are passed up through the graft, using the previously placed suture-loop (left shoulder, view from the anterolateral portal; AA—anterior anchor, PA—posterior anchor, GT—greater tuberosity); (B) Suture tapes are criss-crossed and secured just past the lateral margin of the tuberosity with knotless anchors, providing excellent compression of the graft over the tuberosity footprint. (C) If a small "dog-ear" is noted after lateral graft fixation, a suture preloaded into the lateral-row anchor can be used to tie it down. (D) Model demonstration of graft fixation to the humeral head.

7.7. Anterior and posterior convergence

Once the graft is secured medially and laterally, side-to-side margin convergence sutures are placed to secure the graft to the intact cuff (**Figure 18A** and **B**). Pre-placed sutures are helpful for this, as discussed above. Typically two side-to-side sutures are used posteriorly, to connect the graft to the intact part of the infraspinatus or to the teres minor. Anteriorly, if the fixation is to the intact remaining supraspinatus, two sutures may be used as well (**Figure 18C**); however, if there is no supraspinatus left, and fixation is to the upper border of the subscapularis, no more than one suture should be used, as laterally as possible, to avoid over-constricting the rotator interval. If the distance between the anterior edge of the graft and the upper border of the subscapularis is too great, no margin convergence sutures are placed here.

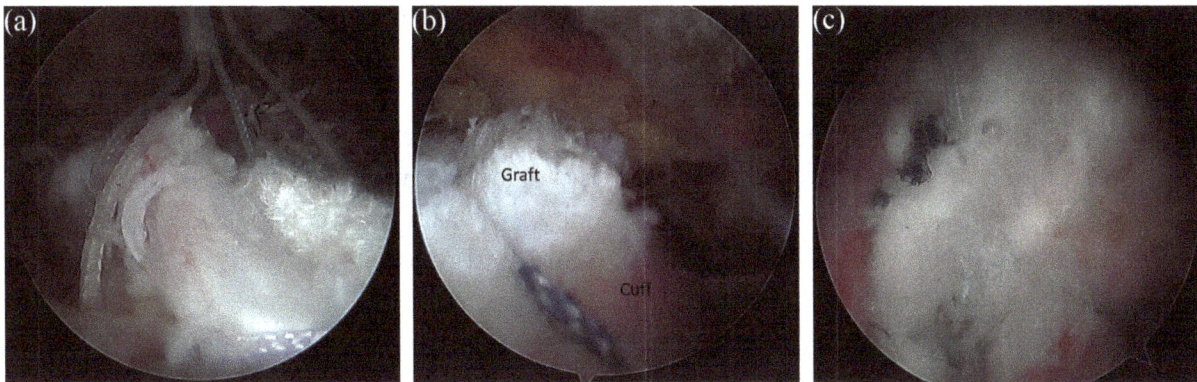

Figure 18. Side-to-side repair to the intact cuff and completion of the SCR. (A) Sutures are passed through the graft and adjacent intact cuff. (B) Sutures are then tied, providing close approximation between the graft and native tissue. (C) Superior view from the Neviaser portal, showing a completed SCR, with excellent coverage of the joint by the graft and native cuff, repaired to the graft.

The shoulder is then taken through a full range of motion to ensure no signs of impingement. And residual spurs on the acromion, or osteophytes off the inferior distal clavicle should be resected (**Figure 8**).

7.8. Postoperative protocol

We follow the same protocol for our SCR cases as for our large rotator cuff repair cases. A shoulder immobilizer sling is worn for 6 weeks, with or without an abduction pillow. Passive range of motion exercises are started at 4–6 weeks postoperatively, active-assisted motion is allowed at 6–8 weeks, and full active motion is allowed after 8 weeks. Strengthening progresses after 12 weeks, and return to activities which require overhead lifting is allowed no earlier than 16 weeks. Typical full return to activities is allowed 6 months postoperatively.

8. Outcomes

Published reports of clinical outcomes following superior capsular reconstruction thus far have been limited to one study, but more such studies are currently either in data collection or already in preparations to report outcomes. In 2013, Mihata et al. reported a case series of 24 shoulders (23 consecutive patients), treated with SCR using fascia lata autograft, with minimum 2-year follow-up [2]. At an average follow-up of 34 months (24–51 months), mean active elevation increased from 84 to 148° and mean external rotation increased from 26 to 40°. All clinical outcomes scores improved significantly, with American Shoulder and Elbow Surgeons score (ASES) score going up from an average of 23.5 to 92.9. Furthermore, imaging showed acromiohumeral distance increased from 4.6 to 8.7 mm, on average. No procedure-related complications were reported [2].

In the United States, most surgeons prefer to use a dermal allograft (Arthrex Arthroflex), which is a thick (3 mm) and durable patch, which requires minimal preparation time and is relatively easy to handle. Several technical reports using this graft have been published, including those by Hirahara and Adams, Petri et al., Tokish and Beicker, and Burkhart et al. [36–39], but clinical data on the outcomes of this approach is lacking in the published literature. However, personal communication with a number of surgeons currently performing SCR using the dermal allograft patch produced reports of high patient satisfaction rates, excellent improvement in function and pain levels in the short term, and low risk of complications. One of our personal communications has been with a surgeon who now has data on 20 SCR procedures, with a minimum follow-up of 3 months and up to 1.5 years, and reports that Visual Analogue Scale (VAS) scores decreased on average from 6–9 to 0–3 range, while ASES scores went up from the 20–30 range to the 70–90 range. No complications were reported in this patient group (personal communication with Dr. Kevin Kaplan, Jacksonville Orthopedic Institute, Jacksonville, FL).

9. Future direction and conclusion

Large irreparable rotator cuff tears in younger and active patients continue to pose a significant clinical challenge to orthopedic surgeons. Arthroplasty treatment option with a reverse shoulder replacement is not ideal in this patient population. Mihata et al. [33] have shown in biomechanical cadaveric studies that a graft reconstruction can restore superior glenohumeral translation when the graft is attached to the glenoid medially and humeral head laterally. However, many technical aspects of this procedure have not been well studied, such as ideal suture and anchor configuration medially or laterally, ideal graft tissue (allograft versus autograft), ideal graft thickness, or ideal tensioning technique.

In the immediate future, we will need larger clinical studies with short, medium, and long-term outcome data demonstrating the effectiveness of superior capsular reconstruction. Radiographic follow-up studies are needed to document graft incorporation or deterioration after this surgery, as well as to monitor the acromiohumeral distance in this patient population. Clinical indications and contraindications, as well as the ideal patient population, for this procedure need be better defined.

Superior capsular reconstruction is a novel technique that may provide a potentially promising solution to a tough problem in the shoulder region. The procedure should be considered for active and physiologically young patients with high functional demand on their upper extremity, and an irreparable rotator cuff tear, and should be performed by surgeons experienced in treating shoulder pathology. More clinical studies are needed before we can advocate widespread use of this procedure in general orthopedic practice.

Author details

Alexander Golant[1]*, Daiji Kano[2], Tony Quach[1], Kevin Jiang[1] and Jeffrey E. Rosen[1]

*Address all correspondence to: alg9067@nyp.org

1 Department of Orthopedics and Rehabilitation, NewYork-Presbyterian Queens, New York City, USA

2 Department of Surgery, NewYork-Presbyterian Queens, New York City, USA

References

[1] Sambandam SN. Rotator cuff tears: An evidence based approach. World J Orthop. 2015;**6**(11):902-918. DOI: 10.5312/wjo.v6.i11.902

[2] Mihata T, Lee TQ, Watanabe C, Fukunishi K, Ohue M, Tsujimura T, Kinoshita M. Clinical results of arthroscopic superior capsule reconstruction for irreparable rotator cuff tears. Arthroscopy. 2013;**29**(3):459-470. DOI: 10.1016/j.arthro.2012.10.022

[3] Tashjian RZ. Epidemiology, natural history, and indications for treatment of rotator cuff tears. Clinics in Sports Medicine. 2012;**31**(4):589-604. DOI: 10.1016/j.csm.2012.07.001

[4] Yadav H, Nho S, Romeo A, Macgillivray JD. Rotator cuff tears: Pathology and repair. Knee Surgery, Sports Traumatology, Arthroscopy. 2009;**17**(4):409-421. DOI: 10.1007/s00167-008-0686-8

[5] Nimura A, Kato A, Yamaguchi K, Mochizuki T, Okawa A, Sugaya H, Akita K. The superior capsule of the shoulder joint complements the insertion of the rotator cuff. Journal of Shoulder and Elbow Surgery. 2012;**21**(7):867-872. DOI: 10.1016/j.jse.2011.04.034

[6] Greene WB, Netter FH. Netter's Orthopaedics. Philadelphia, PA; Saunders Elsevier, 2006

[7] Frank RM, Taylor D, Verma NN, Romeo AA, Mologne TS, Provencher MT. The rotator interval of the shoulder: Implications in the treatment of shoulder instability. Orthopaedic Journal of Sports Medicine. 2015;**3**(12):2325967115621494. DOI: 10.1177/2325967115621494

[8] Jost B, Koch PP, Gerber C. Anatomy and functional aspects of the rotator interval. Journal of Shoulder and Elbow Surgery. 2000;**9**(4):336-341

[9] Burkhart SS, Esch JC, Jolson RS. The rotator crescent and rotator cable: An anatomic description of the shoulder's "suspension bridge". Arthroscopy. 1993;**9**(6):611-616

[10] Ishihara Y, Mihata T, Tamboli M, Nguyen L, Park KJ, Mcgarry MH, Takai S, Lee TQ. Role of the superior shoulder capsule in passive stability of the glenohumeral joint. Journal of Shoulder and Elbow Surgery. 2014;**23**(5):642-648. DOI: 10.1016/j.jse.2013.09.025

[11] Bouaicha S, Slankamenac K, Moor BK, Tok S, Andreisek G, Finkenstaedt T. Cross-sectional area of the rotator cuff muscles in MRI – Is there evidence for a biomechanical balanced shoulder?. PLoS One. 2016;**11**(6):e0157946. DOI: 10.1371/journal.pone.0157946

[12] Eajazi A, Kussman S, LeBedis C, Guermazi A, Kompel A, Jawa A, Murakami AM. Rotator cuff tear arthropathy: Pathophysiology, imaging characteristics, and treatment options. AJR Am J Roentgenol. 2015;**205**(5):W502-W511. DOI: 10.2214/AJR.14.13815

[13] Gumina S, Carbone S, Campagna V, Candela V, Sacchetti FM, Giannicola G. The impact of aging on rotator cuff tear size. Musculoskeletal Surgery. 2013;**97**(Suppl 1):69-72. DOI: 10.1007/s12306-013-0263-2

[14] Abboud JA, Kim JS. The effect of hypercholesterolemia on rotator cuff disease. Clinical Orthopaedics and Related Research. 2010;**468**(6):1493-1497. DOI: 10.1007/s11999-009-1151-9

[15] Thankam FG, Dilisio MF, Agrawal DK. Immunobiological factors aggravating the fatty infiltration on tendons and muscles in rotator cuff lesions. Molecular and Cellular Biochemistry. 2016;**417**(1-2):17-33. DOI: 10.1007/s11010-016-2710-5

[16] Neer CS. Anterior acromioplasty for the chronic impingement syndrome in the shoulder: A preliminary report. J Bone Joint Surg Am. American Volume. 1972;**54**(1):41-50

[17] Bigliani LU, Ticker JB, Flatow EL, Soslowsky LJ, Mow VC. The relationship of acromial architecture to rotator cuff disease. Clinics in Sports Medicine. 1991;**10**(4):823-838

[18] Song L, Miao L, Zhang P, Wang WL. Does concomitant acromioplasty facilitate arthroscopic repair of full-thickness rotator cuff tears? A meta-analysis with trial sequential analysis of randomized controlled trials. SpringerPlus. 2016;**5**(1):685. DOI: 10.1186/s40064-016-2311-5

[19] Kibler WB. Scapular involvement in impingement: Signs and symptoms. Instructional Course Lectures. 2006;**55**:35-43

[20] Jones CK, Savoie FH 3rd. Arthroscopic repair of large and massive rotator cuff tears. Arthroscopy. 2003;**19**(6):564-571

[21] Burkhart SS, Danaceau SM, Pearce CE Jr. Arthroscopic rotator cuff repair: Analysis of results by tear size and by repair technique-margin convergence versus direct tendon-to-bone repair. Arthroscopy. 2001;**17**(9):905-912

[22] Murray TF Jr, Lajtai G, Mileski RM, Snyder SJ. Arthroscopic repair of medium to large full-thickness rotator cuff tears: Outcome at 2- to 6-year follow-up. Journal of Shoulder and Elbow Surgery. 2002;**11**(1):19-24

[23] Wolf EM, Pennington WT, Agrawal V. Arthroscopic rotator cuff repair: 4- to 10-year results. Arthroscopy. 2004;**20**(1):5-12

[24] McElvany MD, McGoldrick E, Gee AO, Neradilek MB, Matsen FA 3rd. Rotator cuff repair: Published evidence on factors associated with repair integrity and clinical outcome. The American Journal of Sports Medicine. 2015;**43**(2):491-500. DOI: 10.1177/0363546514529644

[25] Goutallier D, Postel JM, Bernageau J, Lavau L, Voisin MC. Fatty muscle degeneration in cuff ruptures. Pre- and postoperative evaluation by CT scan. Clinical Orthopaedics and Related Research. 1994;**304**:78-83

[26] Park JS, Park HJ, Kim SH, Oh JH. Prognostic factors affecting rotator cuff healing after arthroscopic repair in small to medium-sized tears. The American Journal of Sports Medicine. 2015;**43**(10):2386-2392. DOI: 10.1177/0363546515594449

[27] Burkhart SS, Nottage WM, Ogilvie-Harris DJ, Kohn HS, Pachelli A. Partial repair of irreparable rotator cuff tears. Arthroscopy. 1994;**10**(4):363-370

[28] Shon MS, Koh KH, Lim TK, Kim WJ, Kim KC, Yoo JC. Arthroscopic partial repair of irreparable rotator cuff tears: Preoperative factors associated with outcome deterioration over 2 years. The American Journal of Sports Medicine. 2015;**43**(8):1965-1975. DOI: 10.1177/0363546515585122

[29] Lewington MR, Ferguson DP, Smith TD, Burks R, Coady C, Wong IH. Graft utilization in the bridging reconstruction of irreparable rotator cuff tears: A systematic review. Am J Sports Med. DOI: 10.1177/0363546517694355. [Epub ahead of print]

[30] Gillespie RJ, Knapik DM, Akkus O. Biologic and synthetic grafts in the reconstruction of large to massive rotator cuff tears. The Journal of the American Academy of Orthopaedic Surgeons. 2016;24(12):823-828

[31] Omid R, Lee B. Tendon transfers for irreparable rotator cuff tears. The Journal of the American Academy of Orthopaedic Surgeons. 2013;21(8):492-501. DOI: 10.5435/JAAOS-21-08-492

[32] Ecklund KJ, Lee TQ, Tibone J, Gupta R. Rotator cuff tear arthropathy. The Journal of the American Academy of Orthopaedic Surgeons. 2007;15(6):340-349

[33] Mihata T, Mcgarry MH, Pirolo JM, Kinoshita M, Lee TQ. Superior capsule reconstruction to restore superior stability in irreparable rotator cuff tears: A biomechanical cadaveric study. The American Journal of Sports Medicine. 2012;40(10):2248-2255

[34] Mihata T, Mcgarry MH, Kahn T, Goldberg I, Neo M, Lee TQ. Biomechanical effect of thickness and tension of fascia lata graft on glenohumeral stability for superior capsule reconstruction in irreparable supraspinatus tears. Arthroscopy. 2016;32(3):418-426. DOI: 10.1016/j.arthro.2015.08.024

[35] Gupta AK, Hug K, Berkoff DJ, Boggess BR, Gavigan M, Malley PC, Toth AP. Dermal tissue allograft for the repair of massive irreparable rotator cuff tears. The American Journal of Sports Medicine. 2012;40(1):141-147. DOI: 10.1177/0363546511422795

[36] Hirahara AM, Adams CR. Arthroscopic superior capsular reconstruction for treatment of massive irreparable rotator cuff tears. Arthroscopy Techniques. 2015;4(6):e637-e641. DOI: 10.1016/j.eats.2015.07.006

[37] Petri M, Greenspoon JA, Millett PJ. Arthroscopic superior capsule reconstruction for irreparable rotator cuff tears. Arthroscopy Techniques. 2015;4(6):e751-e755. DOI: 10.1016/j.eats.2015.07.018

[38] Tokish JM, Beicker C. Superior capsule reconstruction technique using an acellular dermal allograft. Arthroscopy Techniques. 2015;4(6):e833-e839. DOI: 10.1016/j.eats.2015.08.005

[39] Burkhart SS, Adams CR, Denard PJ, Brady PC, Hartzler RU. The arthroscopic superior capsular reconstruction for massive irreparable rotator cuff repair. Arthroscopy Techniques. 2016;5(6):e1407-e1418. DOI: 10.1016/j.eats.2016.08.024

[40] Mihata T, McGarry MH, Kahn T, Goldberg I, Neo M, Lee TQ. Biomechanical effects of acromioplasty on superior capsule reconstruction for irreparable supraspinatus tendon tears. The American Journal of Sports Medicine. 2016;44(1):191-197. DOI: 10.1177/0363546515608652

2

The Role of Physical Medicine and Rehabilitation in Shoulder Disorders

Raoul Saggini, Simona Maria Carmignano,
Lucia Cosenza, Tommaso Palermo and
Rosa Grazia Bellomo

Abstract

Shoulder pain is a common problem and it is responsible for a high proportion of patients presenting to general practice, causing work absenteeism and claims for sickness. A lot of factors and conditions can contribute to shoulder pain. The most prevalent cause is rotator cuff tendinitis; its relevance is correlated not only to its high prevalence rate but also to the fact that is disabling, causing high direct and indirect cost in industrialized country. Other causes of shoulder pain are shoulder impingement syndrome, calcific tendonitis, frozen shoulder, etc. In this context, physical medicine and rehabilitation plays a fundamental role. The conservative approach consists of several interventions. The aim is to decrease shoulder pain and to regain shoulder function, with the goal to reduce the degree of impingement, decreasing swelling and inflammation, and to minimize the risk of further injuries. The purpose of this chapter is to give an overview about shoulder disorders and their conservative treatment by means of physical therapy.

Keywords: shoulder disorders, physical therapy, rehabilitation, rotator cuff, frozen shoulder, ESWT

1. Introduction

Shoulder pain is a widespread problem and is responsible for a high percentage of patients presenting to general practice, causing absenteeism and labor complaints for sickness [1].

A lot of factors and conditions may contribute to shoulder pain. The most common cause is rotator cuff tendinopathy; its importance is linked not only to its high prevalence rate, but also because it is a disabling condition, causing high costs for health service [2].

As mentioned, rotator cuff injury is one of the most common shoulder disorders. Among these, the most common are tendinosis, partial thickness tear, and complete rupture. The incidence of the cuff injuries varies from 5 to 39%; it increases in the elderly population, being approximately 6 and 30%, respectively in patients aged below and above 60 years [3].

In this context, physical medicine and rehabilitation plays a fundamental role. The conservative approach consists of several interventions. The aim of these is to decrease shoulder pain and to regain shoulder function, with the goal to reduce the degree of impingement, decreasing swelling and inflammation, and minimizing the risk of further injuries. Many studies have shown that conservative therapy is the first-line treatment for shoulder disorders, in fact rehabilitative approach allows a reduction in pain feeling and symptoms within few weeks [4].

In literature, several studies have proposed conservative treatment for shoulder diseases, such as non-steroidal anti-inflammatory drugs (NSAIDs), cortisone injections, stretching and strengthening exercises, manual therapy, and physical energies (cryotherapy, extracorporeal shock wave therapy (ESWT), laser therapy, ultrasounds, etc.) to reduce pain feeling and restore shoulder range of motion (ROM) and function.

The purpose of this chapter is to give an overview about shoulder disorders and their conservative treatment by means of physical therapy, reviewing scientific researches, and merging it with our experience in this field. Rehabilitation of shoulder disorders is not easy, because its complex function, which involves not only local structures integrity, but also biomechanics contribution, form other body subsystems. For this reason, it is important to highlight the need of establish a global rehabilitative approach.

2. Biomechanics

Understanding rotator cuff functions and shoulder biomechanics, it is crucial to understand shoulder disorders and their pathogenesis. The rotator cuff allows the stabilization of the glenohumeral joint, compressing the humeral head on the glenoid of the scapula [5, 6]. This mechanism is due to the equal and opposite action of the subscapularis anteriorly and infraspinatus and teres minor muscles posteriorly [7–10].

Scientific studies about shoulder biomechanics have explained precisely the contribution of every ligaments, tendons and muscles to shoulder stability. The action of rotator cuff is to compress the humeral head against scapular glenoid giving stabilization to the joint and allowing concentric rotation [6, 11–13]. Rotator cuff muscles play an important role in stabilizing glenohumeral joint through this compressive mechanism, in particular during mid-ranges motion in which ligaments are lax [14]. Concavity compression mechanism is also important at end-ranges of motion, during which rotator cuff muscles protects ligaments by limiting the range of motion [15, 16] and decreasing strain, usually increased when shoulder reaches maximum abduction and extrarotation [14, 17, 18]. When shoulder joint is in neutral position, rotator cuff muscles contribute equally in providing anterior stability [19]. However, with glenohumeral joint in end-range abduction, subscapularis is a less effective stabilizer than other muscles, while the biceps brachii starts to play a role in joint stability [20].

The "concavity compression" is an important stability mechanism. The compression of the humeral head (convex), exercised by muscles of the rotator cuff, on the glenoid cavity (concave), maintains stable humeral epiphysis, in relation to translational forces. Resistance to joint subluxation is directly proportional to the depth of the articular concavity and to the compression force exerted by the muscles of the rotator cuff [15]. Concavity compression, providing stability of glenohumeral joint, also depends on the extension of glenoid's articular surface (glenoid arc) available to accommodate humeral head [21].

Stabilization function is made evident when the disease is established; in fact, a rotator cuff tear results in the inefficiency of this mechanism with the consequent sliding of the humeral head upward. This is due to the action of the upper fibers of the deltoid muscle, resulting in a subacromial impingement [22].

The action of the rotator cuff muscles must be highly coordinated to be able to perform a specific movement. The muscles must work in coordination, as the rotation of the glen humeral joint does not have a fixed axis [23].

Tension loads acting on rotator cuff tendons can be divided into two types: concentric and eccentric. Concentric ones are generated when humerus has the same direction of cuff muscle, as it happens during abduction against resistance. These loads are better tolerated by the cuff insertion, which clears the acromion at low angles of elevation, protecting it from impingement by the coracoacromial arch. Eccentric tension loads are produced when the arm movement is opposed to the direction of cuff muscles direction. This occurs in example during active resistance to a downward force applied on the humerus. In fact, when the humeral head rotates with respect of the scapula, bending loads stress cuff tendons; cuff elasticity permits to resist these loads. Rotator cuff tendons are also subjected to compressive loads; an upwardly load presses the cuff between the humeral head and the coracoacromial arch [24]. Furthermore, it has demonstrated a morphologic adaptation of the supraspinatus tendon with fibrocartilaginous areas in regions of compression, due to mechanical forces [25].

Every rotator cuff muscle origins on the scapula, which therefore influences the activity of these muscles. Therefore, rotator cuff performance is strictly related to the functional state of the scapula. When this bone is well stabilized, thus presenting the proper position in both static and dynamic tasks, it permits rotator cuff to work at an optimal level. However, alterations in scapular kinematics produce an unstable support to rotator cuff and consequently it affects the biomechanics of the shoulder. Scapular dysfunctions may be causative in rotator cuff disorders or may be the result of rotator cuff injuries, increasing the alteration [26].

Many authors have studied scapula kinematics in patients with rotator cuff diseases; alterations in scapular function have been found in most studies. In subjects with clinical symptoms or imaging demonstrating rotator cuff disorders, studies have demonstrated biomechanics alterations, especially scapular dyskinesia [27]. Possible alterations are not consistent, with various combinations of changes like increase in upward rotation, decrease in posterior tilt and increase in internal rotation. However, the exact relationship between scapular dyskinesia and rotator cuff disorder is not completely clear; is dyskinesis a cause, an effect or a compensation? [26]

3. Shoulder disorders

Pathogenesis of rotator cuff injuries is not completely clear, but it may arise from extrinsic factors, impingement by structures surrounding the cuff, and intrinsic alterations of the tendon itself [28].

On the tendinous portion of the rotator cuff impingement by the coracoacromial ligament and the acromion itself is responsible for the characteristic "impingement syndrome". A peculiar proliferative spur and ridge on the anterior lip and undersurface of the acromial anterior process has been found; furthermore, in many studies this area has shown erosions [4].

Anatomical changes may excessively narrow the subacromial space, in which rotator cuff tendons pass through, and include acromial shape variations (i.e. hooked acromion), orientation of the acromial angle or prominent osseous changes of the inferior portion of the acromion-clavicular joint [29]. In 1986, Bigliani [30] described the important role of acromion shape, as an extrinsic mechanism, in rotator cuff tendinopathy; acromion classified into three types based on different shapes (**Figure 1**): Flat (Type I), Curved (Type II) and Hooked (Type III).

Association between acromion shape and severity of rotator cuff disorder has been well documented, with a greater prevalence of hooked acromion in subjects with subacromial impingement syndrome and full thickness tears. Alterations of shoulder kinematics, postural abnormalities, rotator cuff muscles deficits and decreased extensibility of pectoralis minor are biomechanical factors which can lead to rotator cuff tendons compression [4]. In addition,

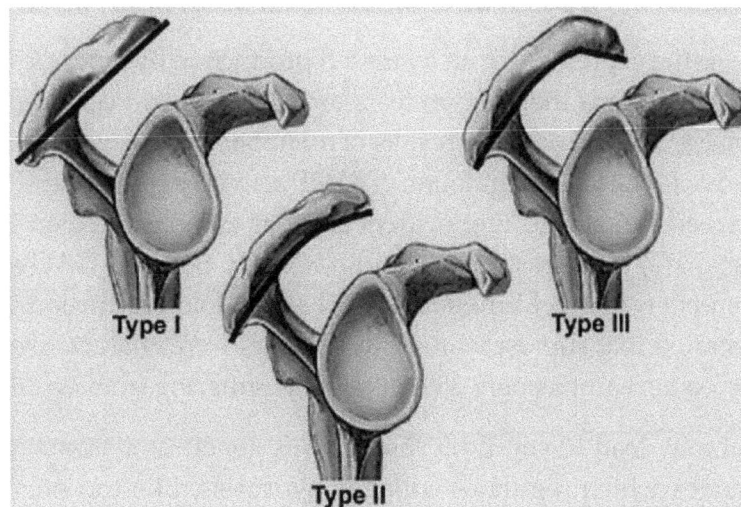

Figure 1. Bigliani classification for acromial in different shapes.

shoulder kinematic alterations can cause a dynamic reduction of the subacromial space (compressing rotator cuff tendons) due to a superior shift of the humeral head [31] or an altered scapula biomechanics that leads acromion sliding downwards [32].

Recent studies suggested that subacromial bursa is a pro-inflammatory membrane responsible for shoulder pain and other subacromial disorders. Blaine [33] demonstrated that inflammatory cytokines, such as Tumor necrosis factor (TNF), Interleukin 1 (IL-1), Interleukin 6 (IL-6), cyclooxygenase-1 (COX-1) and cyclooxygenase-2 (COX-2), increase in subacromial bursal in subjects suffering from bursitis and rotator cuff syndrome. It should also be pointed out that IL-1 and IL-6 play an important role as mediators of collagen catabolism [34].

Peritendinous alterations in rotator cuff disorders are thought to be a secondary phenomenon. Chandler [35] showed that the increased tension in the coracoacromial ligament, due to tendinopathy, stimulates the neoformation of bone on the underside of the acromion, which may result in an impingement syndrome leading to enthesopathy.

Acromial lateral sloping or glenoid version is structural features which play an important role in rotator cuff pathology as extrinsic factors. As mentioned in the previous paragraph, acromion shape influences supraspinatus tendon as it passes under the coracoacromial arch. Even a forward scapula posture, caused by forward head posture and increased kyphosis in combination, can reduce the subacromial space [36].

Intrinsic factors, causing rotator cuff tendinopathy, affect tendon morphology and performance. There is growing evidence in literature supporting the fundamental role of these mechanisms in shoulder disorders.

Intrinsic mechanisms, such as aging processes, poor vascularity and altered biology, lead to tendon degradation also influencing tensile forces and altering loads [37–40].

A reduction in vascular supply of tendons is implicated in rotator cuff tears pathogenesis. In 1934, Codman described for the first time the "critical zone" (1 cm^2 area between the insertion of supraspinatus tendon at greater tubercle and myotendinous junction) which represents the most common site for tendon injury due to its reduced vascularity [4].

Tendon degeneration is the expression of an increased production by tenocytes of metalloproteinase enzymes (MMP); this means that tendon tears are an active and cell-mediated process. The hypothesis is that rotator cuff tears are the results of an imbalance between tendon synthesis and degradation, maybe due to the failed regulation of MMP activity in response of repeated mechanical strains. Tendon degeneration is further evident as it has demonstrated an increase in sulfated glycosaminoglycans (GAG) in supraspinatus tendinosis [41]. Sulfated GAG are associated with acute inflammation and new matrix formation, as well as amyloid production. A study conducted by Cole [42] demonstrated that supraspinatus chronic tears were characterized by 70% amyloid deposition on tendon context, unlike only 25% in patients suffering from acute traumatic injuries.

Another feature that may lead to shoulder disorders is genetics; it seems to be related to the polymorphism of genes which regulates collagen synthesis, like the one found in Achilles tendinopathy. However, this is just a hypothesis since no genes were identified till now as risk factors for rotator cuff diseases [43–45].

Other factors can influence mechanical properties and tensile loads response including tendon geometry, due to collagen fiber alignment. Among tendon alterations, it is important to highlight tendon irregularity and thinning, observed in subjects suffering from degenerative rotator cuff tendinopathy; these conditions influence mechanical properties. Even aging has been observed to be a negative factor for tendon degeneration. Biomechanical studies showed a reduced elasticity and a decreased tensile strength in tendons with aging [4]. Histological studies about rotator cuff tendons showed degenerative changes (calcifications and fibrovascular proliferation) in elderly in comparison to young people, both groups without history of shoulder disorders. Furthermore, aging causes a reduction in total sulfated GAG and proteoglycans in supraspinatus tendon [46].

Other scientific researches demonstrated in elderly people a reduction of type I collagen and an increase in type III, weaker and more irregularly; however there is no consensus in literature whether these changes are related with aging or a secondary consequence of healing processes to repeated microtrauma (or overuse) [47].

An interesting classification is the one developed by Celli [48] that divides the old denomination "shoulder periarthritis" in four clinical presentations, depending on the type, localization and pain:

1. Acute anterior shoulder: where inflammation is limited to the supraspinatus tendon and/ or to the long head of the biceps tendon.

2. Global acute shoulder: pain is acute and inflammation compromised subdeltoid bursa.

3. Chronic anterior shoulder: pain is chronic and localized on the anterior region.

4. Global chronic shoulder: even in this case the pain is chronic, but it affects the whole shoulder.

This classification has the advantage of easy application, but there is no immediate correlation with the cause of degeneration. The most common cause of shoulder pain is an inflammation of the bursae around the glenohumeral joint. The most affected is the subacromial bursa, located between the acromion and the tendons of rotator cuff, but also subdeltoid, subscapularis and subcoracoid bursae may be affected.

Pain is localized on the side of the proximal part of the arm, but it may also extend distally if the inflammatory process involves subdeltoid bursa, which often communicates with the subacromial one. Movements accentuate symptoms, particularly active abduction, that is markedly limited by pain.

3.1. Rotator cuff tendinosis

The incidence of rotator cuff tendinopathy and degenerative tears increases in aging and it is 40% in subjects over 70 years of age [49].

Rotator cuff tendinosis is due to disorganization in collagen fibers morphology and to alterations in tendon ultrastructure. Earlier studies showed histopathological changes associated with rotator cuff tendinosis: tendon fibers thinning and consequently ultrastructural alterations, cellular apoptosis, granulation tissue production and fibro-cartilaginous changes [50, 51]. The risk of progression, which can lead to full tendon rupture, is related to these histopathological changes.

Hyaline and myxoid degeneration, which can affect collagen fibers, already occur in the degenerated tendon. The consequence of this is a reduction in tensile resistance that predisposes the tendon to rupture [4].

In degenerated tendon, healing processes are altered. In fact, the standard composition and structure of the osteotendinous insertion site, with the transition from non-mineralized to mineralized fibrocartilage, is not achieved. The causes of this poor healing process are multifactorial, but correlated to an inadequate and disorganized expression of the cytokines responsible for the formation of the complex structure and composition of the enthesis [52].

Other factors that may influence healing processes are the presence of inflammatory cells in the osteotendinous insertion site and a small number of stem cells in the tendon-bone interface, which hamper physiological scar formation [53].

Healing process occurs in three steps:

Step 1. Inflammatory phase

Step 2. Repairing phase

Step 3. Remodeling phase

An alteration during one of these phases leads to a bad regenerative process. Recent studies demonstrated the importance of the inflammatory phase, during which there is an increase of neutrophils, macrophages and mast cells in rotator cuff lesions in animal and human models. Millar et al. [54] evaluated rotator cuff tendon samples taken by biopsy during repairing phase. They observed significant infiltration of mast cells and macrophages in earlier phase of tendinopathy. Subsequently macrophages produce transforming growth factor-β1 (TGF-β1), which stimulates collagen formation and proteinase activity.

Fibrovascular scar is probably produced during this phase thanks to the action of macrophages. During the repairing phase of healing process, fibroblasts activation determines the expression of various cytokines, such as basic fibroblast growth factor (bFGF), insulin-like growth factor (IGF-1), platelet-derived growth factor-b (PDGF-b), vascular endothelial growth factor (VEGF), bone morphogenic protein-12 (BMP-12), BMP-13 and BMP-14 [4].

3.2. Calcific tendonitis

Calcific tendonitis can be potentially included in the sum of rotator cuff diseases. Its prevalence is estimated between 2.7 and 20% according to radiographies of asymptomatic adults. Usually occurs between the age of 40 and 50, with a higher prevalence in female sex and in sedentary workers. The probability of becoming symptomatic, both acute and chronic, has been estimated to be higher than 50% [52].

A 2009 study conducted by Maugars et al. [53] pointed out that between 7 and 17% of patients suffering from chronic shoulder pain was due to tendon calcification.

Calcific tendonitis is not simply a degenerative disorder, since calcification is not histologically associated with necrosis or tissue damage, but it is a cell-mediated process similar to an incomplete endochondral ossification.

One of the first authors to describe the calcium deposits cycle was Uhthoff [55] who divided it into two phases: a formative and resorptive one. Other authors subdivided the cycle into three phases: pre-calcification (asymptomatic), calcification (impingement) and post-calcification (acute) [56].

A more complete classification divided this cycle into four phases: pre-calcific phase, during which the fibrocartilaginous transformation occurs in the tendon context in a completely asymptomatic manner; formation phase that consists of the deposition of hydroxyapatite crystals within the tendon; re-absorbing phase, characterized by the release of these crystals and finally post calcific recovering phase.

It is therefore evident that there is currently no standardized histological classification for tendon calcifications in literature.

In concern to the radiographic aspects of calcification, many studies converge on Gartner's classification (1993), whereby three kinds of deposits can be identified. Type I refers to a well-defined and dense deposit, type II identifies a well-distinguished but radiotransparent deposit and finally, type III has a radiotransparent structure but with marginal margins [57].

In fact, the classification of the French Arthroscopic Society [58] also identifies three types of calcifications, indicating them with letters A, B and C (**Figure 2**), which reproduce the description of Gartner.

The authors discussed for a long time about the use of radiographic classification both to choose the most appropriate treatment and as an outcome to evaluate its beneficial effect. The fundamental concept is that radiographic classification is not sufficient on its own, but correlation with the clinical data is always necessary [59, 60].

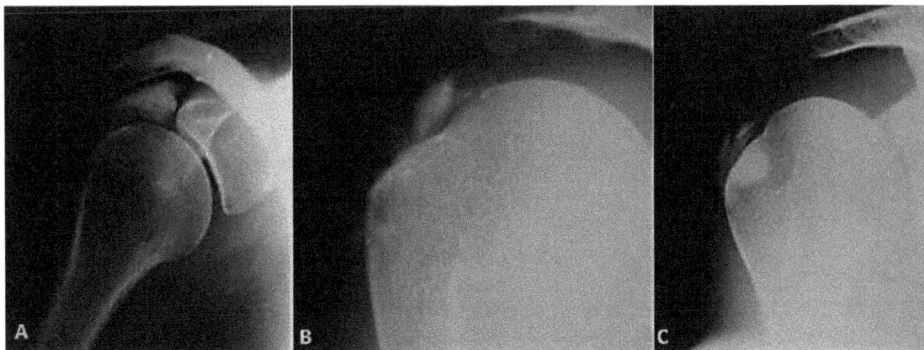

Figure 2. Classification of calcifications by French Arthroscopic Society. A: Dense deposit and well-defined margins, C: nubecular deposit, margins not defined. B: intermediate between the two previous types.

3.3. Subacromial bursitis and impingement

The subacromial bursa is the largest and most complicated bursa in human body. In a 1934 book [61], Codman affirmed that it behaves as a secondary scapula-humeral joint, although it is not composed of cartilage tissue. Therefore, he highlighted the functional issue of subacromial bursa. In 1972, Neer [62] further emphasized this point of view in his studies on impingement syndrome. Moreover, in other studies, he suggested that subacromial bursa is an inflammatory membrane that can lead to pain through nociceptors endings stimulation. Santavirta et al. [63] found a majority of CD-2 and CD-11b mononuclear cells in the bursa of patients suffering from subacromial bursitis. Yanagisawa [64] also demonstrated an increased expression of VEGF in patients with impingement syndrome, thus pointing out chronic inflammation and increased vascularity. Other studies [65] demonstrated the increased expression of pain mediators (substance P) in the subacromial space in subjects with impingement syndrome.

Despite these evidences about subacromial bursa, the changes in biochemical mediators expression, implicated in subacromial impingement syndrome pathogenesis, have not yet completely identified. These investigations were carried on to determine the role of subacromial bursa in impingement syndrome; the question is if the bursa behaves as a pathological or a reparative tissue.

During "bursitis" (**Figure 3**), there is a reduction of the overall subacromial space, which may lead to an increased compression of tissues inside. During subacromial impingement syndrome, it has been demonstrated tendons degeneration, due to inflammatory processes or tension overload in shoulder mobilization (e.g. during work activities) [4].

Impingement syndrome classification was first developed by Neer in 1983 [66] and it is based on histopatological damage of tissues. He defined this syndrome as a mechanical-compressive lesion of tissues of the subacromial space and he identified three progressive stages: first stage ("edema and hemorrhage stage") is typical in patients aged 25 or less with a history of overhead use of the upper limb during sport or work; second stage is defined by further deterioration of rotator cuff tendons and subacromial bursa, and it usually affects 25–40 years old patients; last stage, the third one, is characterized by bone spurs and partial or full-thickness tendon rupture affecting subjects aged 40 or more.

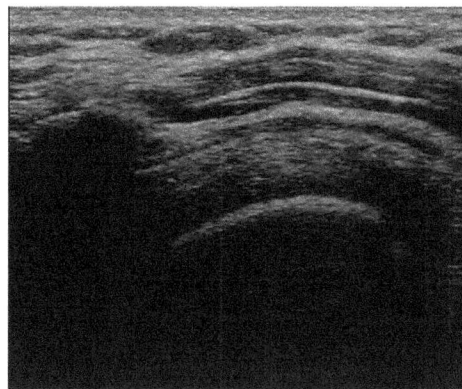

Figure 3. Subacromial bursitis: ultrasound imaging.

3.4. Rotator cuff tears

Rotator cuff tears represent approximately one-third of medical visits for shoulder pain, but sometimes it is a problem difficult to diagnose. Among patients suffering from shoulder pain, rotator cuff tears are the most common cause, especially in subjects aged 60 or more [67]. The incidence of this pathology increases with age; moreover, studies on cadavers have noticed 30% of cases with rotator cuff tears [68]. As mentioned, literature agrees that the incidence increases with age. In particular, a study [69] noted that the incidence of asymptomatic tears in patients aged 50–59 years was 13%, between 60 and 69 years the incidence was 20%, among 70–79 years was 31% and over 80 years was 51%. Yamamoto et al. [67] observed a prevalence of full-thickness tears of 20.7% in a sample population, mean age 57.9 years, with or without symptoms. In a 2006 review of autopsy studies, evaluating 2553 shoulders (mean age 70.1 years), it observed a prevalence of 18.5% for partial-thickness tears and 11.8% for full lesions [68]. Rotator cuff tears are very common, so the pathological history and the clinical examination play a critical role, especially in subclinical cases.

Pathogenesis of rotator cuff tears is complex and multifactorial. For this reason, there are two different schools of thought, according to which tendon injuries can be due to intrinsic or extrinsic factors. Codman [61] had already described the intrinsic theory according to which tendon degenerates in the critical area of hypovascularity; this area is 1 cm from the insertion of supraspinatus to the humeral head. Besides this, due to its low vascularization, it is also an area with low healing capacity. According to extrinsic theory, the cuff tendons, flowing into the subacromial space (i.e. between the acromion, the coracoacromial ligament and the humeral head) can be compressed and then injured.

The majority of rotator cuff tears affected supraspinatus and infraspinatus tendons; these are described as postero-superior cuff tears. On the contrary, antero-superior tears are less common and typically extend anteriorly involving rotator interval or subscapularis tendon. Partial tears consist of a partial disruption of tendon fibers without communication among bursal and articular spaces.

The average normal thickness of rotator cuff tendons is between 8 and 12 mm. The depth of tear defines the degree of lesion. Codman classified tendon tears in three types [61]:

1. bursal-side tear (BT) confined to the bursal surface of the tendon;

2. intratendinous tear (IT), which is localized within tendon thickness and

3. joint-side tear (JT) located on the joint side of the tendon.

Another classification proposed by Neer [62] divided the condition of pain, inflammation, oedema and hemorrhage as stage I, tendinous fibrosis as stage II and fibers rupture as stage III.

Taking into account the average thickness of supraspinatus tendon, Ellman [70] classified rotator cuff tears (**Figure 4**): grade I consists of a tear depth lower than 3 mm (or involving less than 25% of tendon thickness); grade II characterized by a depth between 3 and 6 mm

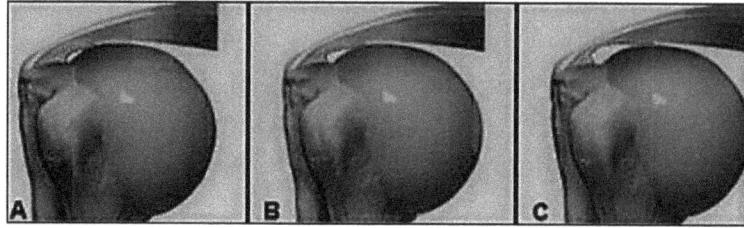

Figure 4. Ellman classification of rotator cuff tears. A: grade I; B: grade II; C: grade III.

or 50% of thickness; grade III involves more than 6 mm or more than 50% of thickness. In full-thickness tears a complete fibers disruption brungs to a direct communication between subacromial and glenohumeral spaces.

Further classifications of rotator cuff tears [4] are shown in **Tables 1–3**.

The greater the size of the lesion, the extent of retraction and the quantity of fatty muscle atrophy, the less the chance of healing from rotator cuff tear. The natural history of the lesion is the further increase in size over time. Therefore, for example, partial thickness tears become total lesions and, referring to Cofield's classification (**Table 1**), small-sized tears tend to evolve toward massive lesions.

3.5. Frozen shoulder

Frozen shoulder, or adhesive capsulitis, is a painful and disabling condition of unknown etiology caused by a spontaneous contracture of the glenohumeral joint in absence of an evident previous event, resulting in reduction of joint motion [71]. This debilitating condition affects from 2 to 5% of the general population [72] and its prevalence increases to 10–38% in patients with comorbidities, such as hypothyroidism [73], diabetes, increased body mass index and cervical spondylosis [74]. This condition is more common in women and in non-dominant shoulders. The mean age of onset is 50–55 years [75].

The currently recognized classification (**Table 4**) identifies as a primary frozen shoulder a condition with any clearly identifiable etiopathogenetic cause, and as secondary a condition triggered by a well-defined cause. The last one, is further subdivided into intrinsic, extrinsic and systemic [76].

Neviaser describe this state as *adhesive capsulitis* to emphasize the inflammatory component affecting the capsule, multiregional areas of synovitis and synovial angiogenesis [77].

Small	<1 cm
Medium	1–3 cm
Large	3–5 cm
Massive	>5 cm

Table 1. Cofield classification (by tear size).

Stage 1	Proximal stump lies close to its bony insertion
Stage 2	Proximal stump retracted at level of humeral head
Stage 3	Proximal stump retracted at glenoid level

Table 2. Patte classification (by cuff tears retraction).

Stage	Muscle description
0	Completely normal muscle
I	Some fatty streaks
II	Amount of muscle is greater than fatty infiltration
III	Amount of muscle is equal to fatty infiltration
IV	Amount of fatty infiltration is greater than muscle

Table 3. Goutallier classification: by extent of fatty muscle degeneration.

Primary adhesive capsulitis	Secondary adhesive capsulitis		
Idiopathic (of unknown etiology or condition)	Systematic • Thyroid disease • Hyperlipidemia • Hypoadrenalism • Chronic obstructive pulmonary disease (COPD) • Osteopenia/reduced bone mineral density • Duputreyn's disease • Ischemic heart conditions • Diabetes mellitus	Extrinsic • Cardiac or breast surgery • Cerebrovascular accident • Cervical radiculopathy	Intrinsic • Impingement • Tendinopathy • Osteoarthritis • Dislocation or shoulder trauma

Table 4. Frozen shoulder classification.

Histological findings attribute to neoangiogenesis the growth of new nerves in the capsuloligamentous complex of these patients and this may be the explanation of the pain associated with capsulitis.

Immunocytochemical analysis on arthroscope biopsy material revealed the presence of chronic inflammatory cells predominantly made up of mast cells, T cells, B cells and macrophages, as well as the presence of fibrosis that results from mast cell infiltrate, which typically regulate the proliferation of fibroblasts [78].

Frozen shoulder seems to be the result of failure of the healing process after an initial inflammatory phase, characterized by an excess of cytokines and growth factors with fibroblasts

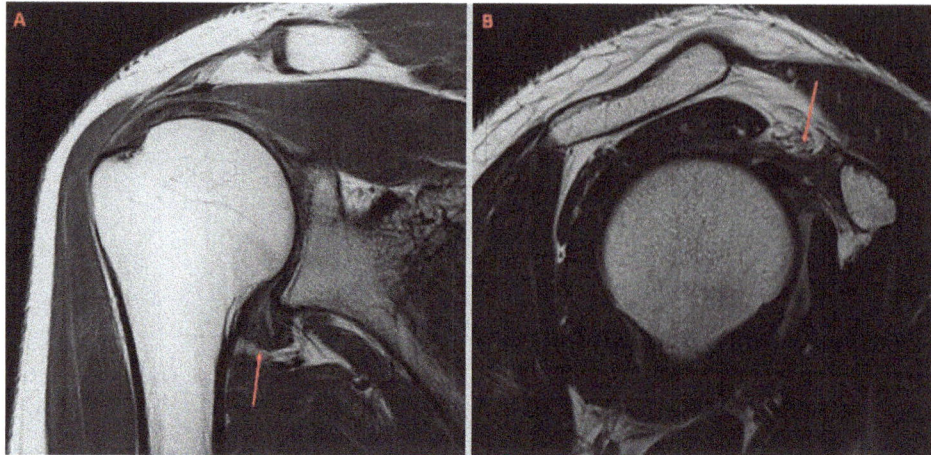

Figure 5. Frozen shoulder at MRI. Coronal PD (A): thickening of the axillary recess of the glenohumeral joint; sagittal PD (B): inflammation in the rotator cuff interval.

accumulation that in part differentiate into myofibroblasts. They exert tractions on new collagen deposits with stiffening of the capsule [79].

The diagnosis is essentially clinical, based on the evidence of the reduction of the ROM (range of motion) in particular in extrarotation, elevation and intrarotation of the glenohumeral joint, in the absence of X-ray lesions. This is accompanied by pain at the insertion of the deltoid and muscular weakness [80]. Radiographic images are not helpful, unless in the case of associated pathologies, such as fractures, arthritis and metallic implants. In selected cases, with suspected association with rotator cuff tendinopathy or impingement syndrome, we can refer to magnetic resonance imaging (**Figure 5**) [81].

According to Neviaser et al. [80], the clinical presentation is indicative of the stage of the adhesive capsulitis:

Stage 1, preadventive stage: patients have mild pain at the end of the range of motion and this condition is often mistakenly diagnosed as impingement syndrome.

Stage 2, "freezing" stage: is often characterized by a high level of discomfort and a high level of pain and a progressive loss of ROM.

Stage 3, "frozen" stage: is characterized by significant stiffness, but less pain.

Stage 4, "thawing" stage: in this phase we have painless stiffness and motion that typically improves by remodeling.

4. Clinical presentation

The diagnosis is based essentially on clinical examination, exclusion of other pathologies and normal glenohumeral radiographs. Initial evaluation of global postural assessment should be perform before focusing on the shoulder, because shoulder pain is often associated with thoracic and cervical spine alignment that alters the scapula's rest position [82]. Postural abnormalities related to shoulder pain, include extension of the atlanto-occipital joints, reduction of physiological cervical lordosis, increase of dorsal kyphosis, protrusion (abduction) of the scapula with rotation downward and internal rotation of the humerus. All these results in neuromusculoskeletal changes.

A thorough collection of the patient's medical history is used to detect if pain origins really from shoulder whether it is a referred pain from other anatomical structures. It is frequently reported that the pain in the shoulder is actually coming from the cervical spine, in which case the irradiation along the upper limb pain, radicular pathology reaches generally until the hand and the fingers, while the pain that starts from the shoulder radiates up and not past the elbow.

The shoulder physical examination can be expressed in the following steps: inspection, palpation, mobility and specific functional tests. The inspection is usually negative, while palpation may aid in the diagnosis. Palpation should include all the articulation of the scapular girdle and all the rotator cuff muscles trying to overcome with appropriate maneuvres the deltoid that covers a large part of the rotator cuff. During the palpation, must be taken simultaneously consider several aspects. They are: the tenderness, the swelling, changes in temperature, the deformity, both obvious and hidden, the muscle characteristics and the relations between the various structures. The motion of both shoulders should be assessed actively and passively. Forward elevation and elevation in the scapular plane as well as internal and external rotation with the arm at the side and in 90° of abduction should be performed.

Tests of affected muscles against resistance are imperative to formulate a correct diagnosis.

Neer test: the doctor is placed behind the patient, with one hand passively he raises his arm in internal rotation and abduction, while with the other stabilizes the scapula. If the patient refers pain in an arc of movement between 70° and 120°, the test shows a conflict between the greater tuberosity and the humeral the acromion.

Hawkins test: it is performed with arm at 90° of flexion front and elbow flexed to 90°; in this position the physician, in front of the patient and imprints an internal rotational movement of the glenohumeral joint. Pain located below the acromioclavicular joint with internal rotation is considered a positive test result and it is indicative of inflammation of the subacromial bursa or of an impingement of all structures that are located between the greater tubercle of the humerus and the coracohumeral ligament.

Palm-up test: the examiner contrasts the movement of the patient to elevate the arm with the elbow in extension and palm of the hand facing up. If the test shows pain is positive to a lesion of the long head of the humeral biceps.

Jobe test: the examiner stands in front of the patient keeps his arms positioned at 90° of abduction, 30° of anterior flexion and maximum intra-rotation (thumbs pointing to the ground). The examiner lowers arms against the patient's resistance against exerting a downward thrust. The test is positive for the supraspinatus muscle if the affected limb is lowered, regardless of whether or not the presence of pain.

Other tests can be used, such as Yocum test, the horizontal adduction test, the painful arc sign, the empty can test, the drop arm test, the Speed test, the Yergason test and the Pattes test.

Clinical evaluation can completed with assessment scales like Constant-Murley scale [83, 84] or simple shoulder test (SST).

The Constant-Murley score is an ordinal scale used in all pathologies of shoulder (not only for the instability), with a score ranging from 0 to 100 (100 = normal shoulder). The scale investigates four areas through the pain (15 points), activities of daily living (20 points), strength (25 points) and the range of motion (40 points). In this way it achieved a full assessment of the level of pain and disability related to the activities of daily living.

The "simple shoulder test" (SST) is a binary scale used for all shoulder pathologies that involves the administration of 12 questions to the patient (normal score = 12). The questions are used to assess the perceived pain and the ability to perform certain activities of daily living. The DASH is halfway between a generic test (as the Short Form) and a specific test for the shoulder, it can use to complete the assessment.

Imaging studies are commonly used to identify and differentiate the source of the injury.

5. Conservative approach

The conservative approach avails of different kind of treatments, whose main purpose is to reduce pain and other signs of inflammation, recover function and prevent further joint damage [85].

A great number of studies support the conservative approach as the main treatment for the mildest forms of shoulder pain due to adhesive capsulitis [86]. The natural course of the frozen shoulder leads to healing in more or less long times. To reduce pain faster and recover the articular functionality, we can intervene with several alone or combined therapies, such as physical therapy (ultrasound, lasers, hyperthermia, electro-analgesia and shock waves), intra-articular corticosteroid injection, intra-articular saline hydrodilation with distention and eventual rupture of the glenohumeral joint capsule, intra-articular sodium hyaluronate injection into the glenohumeral joint, suprascapular nerve block, shoulder manipulation under anesthesia, oral corticosteroid or NSAIDs (non-steroidal anti-inflammatory drugs) and analgesics. In case of failure of these therapies, the alternative is to proceed with open or arthroscopic synovectomy and glenohumeral capsular releases [87–89].

5.1. Extracorporeal shock wave therapy

Since 1980, the extracorporeal impact waves have been used in different conditions, initially to destroy kidney stones. Investigating the side effects on the surrounding tissues, it was understood that they could also find use in the treatment of musculoskeletal disorders [90]. The effect on these tissues is dose-dependent: high doses tend to have destructive effects, low doses have regenerative effects [91].

All the principles that led the application of the ESWT since 1995 have been revised in a recent review, that has established new ones. The recommended energy limit should be beneath 0.28 mJ/mmq, above which necrotic effects prevail; ESWT is performed without anesthesia, even on larger areas; their application also on open growth plates seems to be safe [92].

The regenerative effect of ESWT is the consequence of the activation of gene expression for growth factors or cytokines and fibroblast proliferation. Mechanical stimulation is converted by tendon tissue in enhancement of TGF-β1 gene expression and increase of collagen I and collagen III [93].

The phenomenon of mechanosensing is particularly clear in bone tissue, due to its structure and physiology: it acts like a piezoelectric. After ESWT exposure, bone shows: osteogenic differentiation of mesenchymal stem cells [94]; expression of nitric oxide synthase (eNOS), vascular endothelial growth factor (VEGF) that lead to neoangiogenesis and accelerate tissue regeneration and healing [95]; bone regeneration, starting from periosteum stimulation [96]; direct stimulation of osteoblasts and indirect reduction of osteoclasts activity [97].

In addition, the increase in NOS appears to be involved in another signaling pathway leading to the reduction of pro-inflammatory factors. It has been seen that NOS exerts an inhibitory action on nuclear factor kappa-light-chain-enhancer of activated B cells (NF-κB), hence the role in production of proinflammatory cytokine and leukocytes recruitment, generating pain and phlogosis, are blocked [98].

Other mechanism is the production of NO and VEGF resulting in neoangiogenesis (**Figure 6**) that improves blood supply promoting tissue repairing and wash-out of algogenic and noxious substances [99].

ESWT intervene in pain modulation also by release of endogenous analgesic sustances P and calcitonine gene-related peptide (CGRP) and according to the gate control [100]. About the gate control, Saggini et al. [101], claim that a hyperstimulation-like shock waves, activate the descending inhibitory system, blocking following nociceptive stimuli in the posterior column of the spinal cord. In addition, ESWT modify substances P and CGRP levels, damaging peripheral small unmyelinated fibers, responsible of immediate release of the algogenic peptide. All these mechanisms make ESWT suitable to treat various musculoskeletal disorders, such as calcific tendonitis, epicondylitis, osteoarthritis and long bone fracture [102].

ESWT has proved to be a valid option in the treatment of calcifying tendinitis of the shoulder. A study based on a meta-analysis showed the power of ESWT to intervene in case of calcific

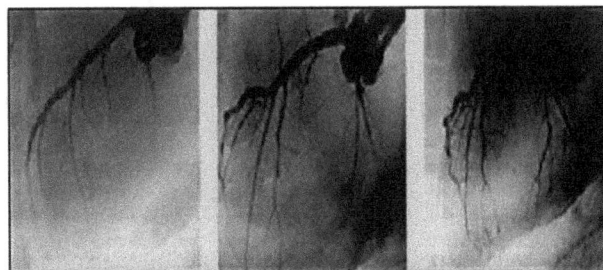

Figure 6. Coronary neovascularization after 4 weeks of shock wave therapy.

tendinitis, promoting resorption of the calcifications using high energy density (conventional limit set at 0.20 mJ/mmq, less than this intensity was labeled low-energy). Functional outcome (Constant-Murley score) and radiographic resorption (chance of complete resorption) of the deposits after 3 months, showed that high-energy ESWT is more effective than low-energy ESWT [103]. The effect on calcifications is not merely mechanical as in the case of kidney stones, but rather biochemical induces interstitial and extracellular changes, enhancing tissue regeneration [104].

Few studies specifically address the application of ESWT in frozen shoulder. One of the study [105], recruited 36 patients divided into 2 groups: one received shock waves (1200 shocks with energy between 0.1 and 0.3 mJ/mmq) and one sham. Pain and disability score were assessed with the Shoulder Pain and Disability Index (SPADI) questionnaire before and after the therapy, and 2 and 5 months after the treatment. The results show a positive effect on recovery of frozen shoulder that was faster than sham group.

Another research [106] compare ESWT (1000 shock waves, with energy between 0.01 and 0.16 mJ/mmq) with conservative physical therapy, both group treated twice a week for six weeks. Pain and function were assessed, respectively, with visual analogue scale (VAS) and patient-specific functional scales (PSFS). Both group showed significant decreases in VAS and PSFS, the ESWT group reported lower score then the control group.

ESWT is therefore a possible way to treat the frozen shoulder, especially if we consider the fact that it is a safe, non-invasive and low cost procedure.

5.2. Intra-articular injections

Intra-articular drug administration offers several advantages: increased bioavailability, reduced systemic effects and fewer side effects. Moreover, most joints can be accessed accurately, especially under ultrasound guidance [107].

Intra-articular injections into the glenohumeral joint are commonly performed to treat different conditions affecting this articulation, such as osteoarthritis, adhesive capsulitis and rheumatoid arthritis. Despite the widespread use of this treatment, there are no standard criteria for their performance [26].

With regard to this type of therapy applied to the treatment of shoulder pain, two substances are used: corticosteroids and hyaluronic acid [108]. The pharmacological properties of corticosteroids are well known, in accordance with them, this procedure is recommended in the acute phase. The risks associated with corticosteroid injection are limited if performed by experienced hands and in patients eligible for such procedure. Injection should be avoided in patients with septic arthritis, bacteremia and in immunocompromised patients [109].

The main purpose in treating the frozen shoulder is to reduce the loss of function and to give relief to pain that significantly limits movement. In the case of adhesive capsulitis, intra-articular administration of corticosteroids is generally associated with conventional physical therapy. A systematic review of 25 studies from 1947 to present, compares infiltrations with manipulation under anesthesia, physical therapy and distension of the joint capsule. In all cases it is clear that intra-articular administration of corticosteroids improves and accelerate patients' healing. Long-term results about conventional therapies versus corticosteroids are comparable; due to understandable considering that adhesive capsulitis is a self-limiting pathology [110].

Another possible application of corticosteroids involves infiltration within the subacromial bursa; this method (**Figure 7**) is particularly useful in those cases of acute painful bursitis, in combination with other therapies aimed at treating the underlying cause.

Besides the corticosteroids, whose action and effectiveness are widely dealt in literature, the use of the viscosupplementation with hyaluronic acid is becoming increasingly widespread [111]. Hyaluronic acid acts through different mechanisms when injected into the joint. It is an anionic, nonsulfated glycosaminoglycan distributed widely throughout connective, epithelial and neural tissues, is capable of retaining water and this contributes to cell adhesion, proliferation and migration. High local concentrations cause the release of growth factors, accelerating the tissue repair process [112]. The viscosupplementation is a way to restore rheological properties of the synovial fluid, enhancing viscoelastic properties of synovial fluid protecting cartilage from mechanical stress and reducing pain [113, 114].

In the tendinitis involving the rotator cuff, viscosupplementation, not only protects the joint surface, but also restores the homeostasis of the chondrocytes [115]. The hypothesis that hyaluronic acid also acts on pain modulation has been investigated and Mitsui et al. [116] demonstrate that hyaluronic acid inhibits not only expression of mRNA for proinflammatory cytokines, such as IL-1b, IL-6 and TNF-a, but also COX-2/PGE2 (Prostaglandin E2) production via CD44 in IL-1-stimulated subacromial-synovium fibroblasts. CD44 is also present on synoviocytes, so it is a target for pain reduction. The restoration of the viscoelastic barrier around the nociceptive afferent fibers, reduces pain, hindering interaction with nociceptive stimuli [117].

5.3. Rehabilitation

The rehabilitation program should always start from clinical evaluation, focusing on the status of functional deficiency, the range of motion and the pain elicited during evaluation [118]. The aim is to ensure long-term results in joint mobility, to reduce stiffness and improve function [119].

Maintaining the range of movements is essential to prevent adhesion and decrease impingement. To intervene on the strength of the rotator cuff muscles and on the scapula stabilizing muscles (anterior serratus, rhomboids, latissimus dorsi and trapezium) and the deltoid,

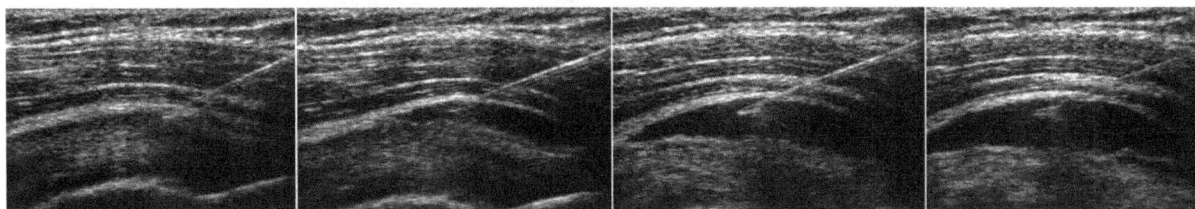

Figure 7. Sequence of subacromial bursa infiltration.

avoids the superior migration of the humeral head and the scapular instability, two conditions that occur in the impingement syndrome.

A deficit in neuromuscular control may cause abnormalities in the rotator cuff and scapula-thoracic muscles. It has been postulated that proprioception can modulate the sensitivity of muscle spindles and help subjects to pay more attention to joint position [120].

Exercises that specifically generate higher level of activation of the rotator cuff, lower trapezius or serratus anterior, are open-chain exercises included full can, side lying external rotation, diagonal exercise and prone full can at 100° of abduction [121]. While the closed-chain exercises facilitate the co-contraction of shoulder muscles as well as strengthen the serratus anterior [122].

The brain guides motion tasks by interacting with external signals and proprioceptive stimuli. Therefore, stimuli integration takes place here and the center that generates an answer to them can be re-edited.

A possible way to reach this aim is the Multi-Joint System® (MJS), a system consisting of a multi-articulated arm run by the patient on the three planes of space (**Figure 8**). The patient receives feedback from a computer system connected to the robot arm and adjusts his movements, following predefined trajectories. In this way, the patient learns to perform all the

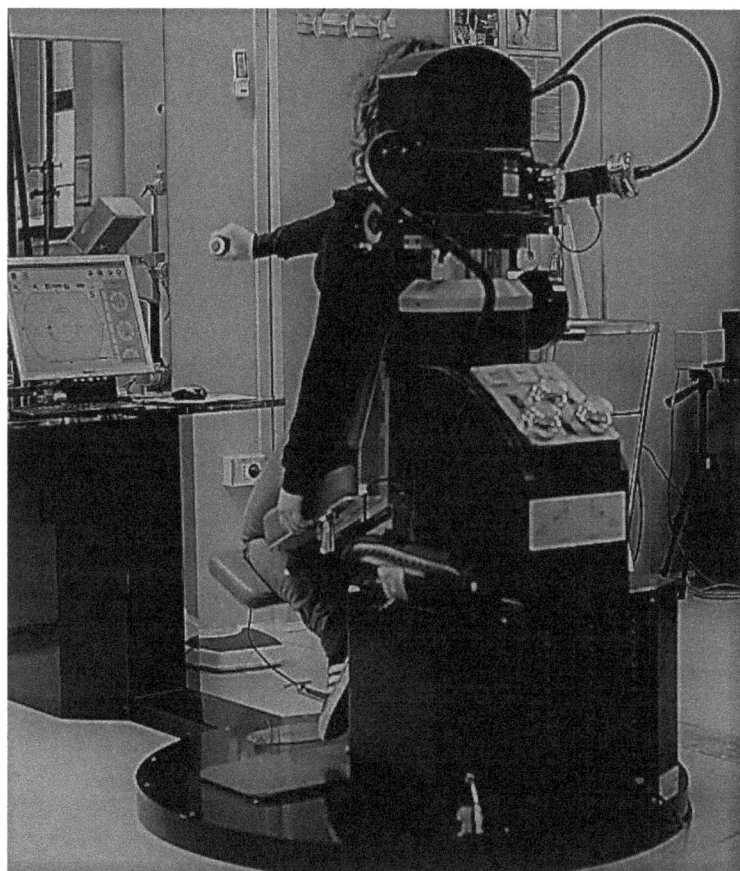

Figure 8. Multi-Joint System®.

peculiar movements of the glenohumeral joint, maintaining a proper position of the scapula and increasing the strength of the anterior serratus, rhomboid, latissimus dorsi, trapezius and deltoid. MJS grant a better control of shoulder movements with increased proprioception, sensitivity and shoulder joint motion in a multi-dimensional axial-type range [123, 124].

Author details

Raoul Saggini[1]*, Simona Maria Carmignano[2], Lucia Cosenza[2], Tommaso Palermo[2] and Rosa Grazia Bellomo[3]

*Address all correspondence to: saggini@unich.it

1 Department of Medical Oral and Biotechnological Sciences, School of Specialty in Physical and Rehabilitation Medicine, "Gabriele d'Annunzio" University, Chieti, Italy

2 School of Specialty in Physical and Rehabilitation Medicine, "Gabriele d'Annunzio" University, Chieti, Italy

3 Physical and Rehabilitation Medicine, Department of Medical Oral and Biotechnological Sciences, "Gabriele d'Annunzio" University, Chieti, Italy

References

[1] Clement ND, Nie YX, McBirnie JM. Management of degenerative rotator cuff tears: A review and treatment strategy. Sports Medicine, Arthroscopy, Rehabilitation, Therapy & Technology. 2012;**4**:48

[2] Sher JS, Uribe JW, Posada A, Murphy BJ, Zlatkin MB. Abnormal findings on magnetic resonance images of asymptomatic shoulders. Journal of Bone and Joint Surgery (American). 1995;**77**:10-15

[3] Tempelhof S, Rupp S, Seil R. Age-related prevalence of rotator cuff tears in asymptomatic shoulders. Journal of Shoulder and Elbow Surgery. 1999;**8**:296-299

[4] Berhart LV, editor. Advances in Medicine and Biology. New York: Nova Science Publisher Inc; 2016. 129-178 p

[5] Bassett RW, Browne AO, Morrey BF, An KN. Glenohumeral muscle force and moment mechanics in a position of shoulder instability. Journal of Biomechanics. 1990;**23**:405-415

[6] Karduna AR, Williams GR, Williams JL, Iannotti JP. Kinematics of the glenohumeral joint: Influences of muscle forces, ligamentous constraints and articular geometry. Journal of Orthopaedic Research. 1996;**14**:986-993

[7] Lippitt S, Matsen F. Mechanisms of glenohumeral joint stability. Clinical Orthopaedics and Related Research. 1993;**291**:20-28

[8] Soslowsky LJ, Carpenter JE, Bucchieri JS, Flatow EL. Biomechanics of the rotator cuff. Orthopedic Clinics of North America. 1997;**28**:17-30

[9] Wuelker N, Roetman B, Plitz W, Knop C. Function of the supraspinatus muscle in a dynamic shoulder model. Unfallchirurg. 1994;**97**:308-313

[10] Sharkey NA, Marder RA, Hanson PB. The entire rotator cuff contributes to elevation of the arm. Journal of Orthopaedic Research. 1994;**12**:699-708

[11] Howell SM, Galinat BJ, Renzi AJ, et al. Normal and abnormal mechanics of the glenohumeral joint in the horizontal plane. Journal of Bone and Joint Surgery (American). 1988;**70**:227-232

[12] Kelkar R, Wang VM, Flatow EL, et al. Glenohumeral mechanics: A study of articular geometry, contact and kinematics. Journal of Shoulder and Elbow Surgery. 2001;**10**:73-84

[13] Poppen NK, Walker PS. Normal and abnormal motion of the shoulder. Journal of Bone and Joint Surgery (American). 1976;**58**:195-201

[14] Howell SM, Kraft TA. The role of the supraspinatus and infraspinatus muscles in glenohumeral kinematics of anterior shoulder instability. Clinical Orthopaedics and Related Research. 1991;**263**:128-134

[15] Lippett S, Vanderhoof J, Harris SL, et al. Glenohumeral stability from concavity-compression: A quantitative analysis. Journal of Shoulder and Elbow Surgery. 1993;**2**:27-34

[16] Neviaser RJ, Neviaser TJ, Neviaser JS. Anterior dislocation of the shoulder and rotator cuff rupture. Clinical Orthopaedics and Related Research. 1993;**291**:103-106

[17] Apreleva M, Parsons IM, Pfaeffe J, et al. 3-D joint reaction forces at the glenohumeral joint during active motion. Advanced Bioengineering. 1998;**39**:33-34

[18] Parsons IM, Apreleva M, Fu FH, et al. The effect of rotator cuff tears on reaction forces at the glenohumeral joint. Journal of Orthopaedic Research. 2002;**20**:439-446

[19] Blaiser RB, Guldberg MS, Rothman ED. Anterior shoulder stability: Contributions of rotator cuff forces and the capsular ligaments in a cadaver model. Journal of Shoulder and Elbow Surgery. 1992;**1**:140-150

[20] Itoi E, Newman SR, Kuechle DK, et al. Dynamic anterior stabilizers of the shoulder with the arm in abduction. Journal of Bone and Joint Surgery (British). 1994;**76**:834-836

[21] Lee SB, Kim KJ, O'Driscoll SW, et al. Dynamic glenohumeral stability provided by the rotator cuff muscles in the mid-range and end-range of motion: A study in cadavera. Journal of Bone & Joint Surgery. 2000;**82**:849-857

[22] Harryman DT 2nd, Sidles JA, Clark JM, McQuade KJ, Gibb TD, Matsen FA 3rd. Translation of the humeral head on the glenoid with passive glenohumeral motion. Journal of Bone and Joint Surgery (American). 1990;**72**:1334-1343

[23] Rowlands LK, Wertsch JJ, Primack SJ, Spreitzer AM, Roberts MM. Kinesiology of the empty can test. American Journal of Physical Medicine & Rehabilitation. 1995;**74**:302-304

[24] Sigholm G, Styf J, Korner L, Herberts P. Pressure recording in the subacromial bursa. Journal of Orthopaedic Research. 1988;74:302-304

[25] Okuda Y, Gorski JP, An KN, Amadio PC. Biochemical, histological, and biomechanical analyses of canine tendon. Journal of Orthopaedic Research. 1987;5:60-68

[26] Maffulli N, editor. Rotator Cuff Tear. Basel: Karger; 2012. 10-17, 27-29, 41-45, 90-93 p

[27] McClure P, Michener LA, Karduna AR. Shoulder function and three-dimensional scapular kinematics in people with and without shoulder impingement syndrome. Physical Therapy. 2006;86:1075-1090

[28] Maffulli N, Longo UG, Gougoulias N, Loppini M, Denaro V. Long-term health outcomes of youth sports injuries. British Journal of Sports Medicine. 2010;44:21-25

[29] Gill TJ, McIrvin E, Kocher MS, Homa K, Mair SD, Hawkins R. The relative importance of acromial morphology and age with respect to rotator cuff pathology. Journal of Shoulder and Elbow Surgery. 2002;11:327-330

[30] Bigliani LU, Morrison DS, April EW. The morphology of the acromion and its relationship to rotator cuff tears. The Journal of Orthopaedic Translation. 1986;10:228

[31] Keener JD, Wei AS, Kim HM, Steger-May K, Yamaguchi K. Proximal humeral migration in shoulders with symptomatic and asymptomatic rotator cuff tears. Journal of Bone and Joint Surgery (American). 2009;91:1405-1413

[32] Ludewig PM, Cook TM. Alterations in shoulder kinematics and associated muscle activity in people with symptoms of shoulder impingement. Physical Therapy. 2000;80:276-291

[33] Blaine TA, Cote MA, Proto A. Interleukin-1β stimulates stromal-derived factor-1α expression in human subacromial bursa. Journal of Orthopaedic Research. 2011;29:1695-1699

[34] Gotoh M, Hamada K, Yamakawa H. Interleukin-1-induced subacromial synovitis and shoulder pain in rotator cuff diseases. Rheumatology (Oxford). 2001;40(9):995-1001

[35] Chandler TJ. Shoulder strength, power, and endurance in college tennis players. The American Journal of Sports Medicine. 1992, July;20:455-458

[36] Solem-Bertoft E, Thuomas KA, Westerberg CE. The influence of scapular retraction and protraction on the width of the subacromial space: An MRI study. Clinical Orthopaedics and Related Research. 1993;296:99-103

[37] Biberthaler P, et al. Microcirculation associated with degenerative rotator cuff lesions. In vivo assessment with orthogonal polarization spectral imaging during arthroscopy of the shoulder. Journal of Bone and Joint Surgery (American). 2003;85-A:475-480

[38] Goodmurphy CW, Osborn J, Akesson EJ, Johnson S, Stanescu V, Regan, WD. Immunocytochemical analysis of torn rotator cuff tendon taken at the time of repair. Journal of Shoulder and Elbow Surgery. 2003;12:368-374

[39] Rudzki JR, et al. Contrast-enhanced ultrasound characterization of the vascularity of the rotator cuff tendon: Age- and activity-related changes in the intact asymptomatic rotator cuff. Journal of Shoulder and Elbow Surgery. 2008;**17**:96S-100S

[40] Huang CY, Wang VM, Pawluk RJ, Bucchieri JS, Levine WN, Bigliani LUJ. Inhomogeneous mechanical behavior of the human supraspinatus tendon under uniaxial loading. Journal of Orthopaedic Research. 2005;**23**:924-930

[41] Seitz AL, McClure PW, Finucane S, Boardman ND, Michener LA. Mechanisms of rotator cuff tendinopathy: Intrinsic, extrinsic, or both? Clinical Biomechanics. 2011;**26**:1-12

[42] Cole AS, Cordiner-Lawrie S, Carr AJ, Athanasou NA. Localised deposition of amyloid in tears of the rotator cuff. The Journal of Bone and Joint Surgery. 2001;**83**(4):561-564

[43] Harvie P, Ostlere SJ, Teh J, McNally EG, Clipsham K, Burston BJ. Genetic influences in the aetiology of tears of the rotator cuff. Sibling risk of a fullthickness tear. Journal of Bone and Joint Surgery (British). 2004;**86**:696-700

[44] Mokone GG, Gajjar M, September AV, Schwellnus MP, Greenberg J, Noakes TD. The guanine–thymine dinucleotide repeat polymorphism within the tenascin-C gene is associated with achilles tendon injuries. The American Journal of Sports Medicine. 2005;**33**:1016-1021

[45] September AV, Schwellnus MP, Collins M. Tendon and ligament injuries: The genetic component. British Journal of Sports Medicine. 2007;**41**:241-246

[46] Rees JD, Maffulli N, Cook J. Management of tendinopathy. The American Journal of Sports Medicine. 2009;**37**(9):1855-1867

[47] Bank RA, TeKoppele JM, Oostingh G, Hazleman BL, Riley GP. Lysylhydroxylation and non-reducible crosslinking of human supraspinatus tendon collagen: Changes with age and in chronic rotator cuff tendinitis. Annals of the Rheumatic Diseases. 1999;**58**:35-41

[48] Celli L, editor. The Shoulder: Periarticular Degenerative Pathology. Vol. 1. Springer, Austria; 1990

[49] Maffulli N, Wong J, Almekinders LC. Types and epidemiology of tendinopathy. Clinics in Sports Medicine. 2003;**22**:675-692

[50] Millar NL, Wei AQ, Molloy TJ, Bonar F, Murrell GA. Cytokines and apoptosis in supraspinatus tendinopathy. Journal of Bone and Joint Surgery (British). 2009, Mar;**91**(3):417-424

[51] Harwood FL, Goomer RS, Gelberman RH, Silva MJ, Amiel D. Regulation of alpha(v) beta3 and alpha5beta1 integrin receptors by basic fibroblast growth factor and platelet-derived growth factor-BB in intrasynovial flexor tendon cells. Wound Repair and Regeneration. 1999;**7**:381-388

[52] Speed CA, Hazleman BL. Calcific tendinitis of the shoulder. The New England Journal of Medicine. 1999;**340**(20):1582-1584

[53] Maugars Y, Varin S, Gouin F, et al. Treatment of shoulder calcifications of the cuff: A controlled study. Joint, Bone, Spine. 2009;**76**(4):369-377

[54] Millar NL, Hueber AJ, Reilly JH, et al. Inflammation is present in early human tendinopathy. The American Journal of Sports Medicine. 2010;**38**(10):2085-2091

[55] Uhthoff HK, Loehr JW. Calcific tendinopathy of the rotator cuff: Pathogenesis, diagnosis, and management. The Journal of the American Academy of Orthopaedic Surgeons. 1997;**5**:183-191

[56] Rowe CR. Calcific tendinitis. Instructional Course Lectures. 1985;**34**:196-198

[57] Gartner J. Tendinosis calcarea—Behandlungsergebnisse mit dem Needling. Zeitschrift Fu r Orthopa die Und Ihre Grenzgebiete. 1993;**131**(5):461-469

[58] Clavert P, Sirveaux F. Les tendinopathies calcifiantes de l'épaule. Revue de Chirurgie Orthopédique et Traumatologique. 2008;**94**(8s):336-355

[59] Serafini G, Sconfienza LM, Lacelli F, Silvestri E, Aliprandi A, Sardanelli F. Rotator cuff calcific tendonitis: Short-term and 10-year outcomes after two-needle US-guided percutaneous treatment-nonrandomized controlled trial. Radiology. 2009;**252**(1):157-164

[60] Ogon P, Suedkamp NP, Jaeger M, Izadpanah K, Koestler W, Maier D. Prognostic factors in nonoperative therapy for chronic symptomatic calcific tendinitis of the shoulder. Arthritis & Rheumatology. 2009;**60**(10):2978-2984

[61] Codman EA, editor. The Shoulder. Boston: Thomas Todd; 1934. 123-215 p

[62] Neer CS. Anterior acromioplasty for the chronic impingement syndrome in the shoulder. Journal of Bone and Joint Surgery (American). 1972;**87**:1399

[63] Santavirta S, Konttinen Y, Antti-Poika I, Nordström D. Inflammation of the subacromial bursa in chronic shoulder pain. Archives of Orthopaedic and Traumatic Surgery. 1992;**111**:336-340

[64] Yanagisawa K, Hamada K, Gotoh MT. Vascular endothelial growth factor (VEGF) expression in the subacromial bursa is increased in patients with impingement syndrome. Journal of Orthopaedic Research. 2001;**19**:448-455

[65] Gotoh M, Hamada K, Yamakawa H, Inoue A, Fukuda H. Increased substance P in subacromial bursa and shoulder pain in rotator cuff diseases. Journal of Orthopaedic Research. 1998;**16**(5):618-621

[66] Neer CS. Impingement lesions. Clinical Orthopaedics and Related Research. 1983;**173**:70-77

[67] Yamamoto A, Takagishi K, Osawa T, Yanagawa T, Nakajima D, Shitara H. Prevalence and risk factors of a rotator cuff tear in the general population. Journal of Shoulder and Elbow Surgery. 2010;**19**:116-120

[68] Reilly P. Dead man and radiologists don't lie: A review of cadaveric and radiological studies of rotator cuff tear prevalence. Annals of the Royal College of Surgeons of England. 2006;**88**:116-121

[69] Ciccotti MA, Ciccotti MC, Ciccotti MG. Rotator cuff injury. Current Sports Medicine Reports. 2009;**8**:52-58

[70] Ellman H. Diagnosis and treatment of incomplete rotator cuff tears. Clinical Orthopaedics and Related Research. 1990;(254):64-74

[71] Cadogan A, Mohammed KD. Shoulder pain in primary care: Frozen shoulder. Journal of Primary Health Care. 2016;**8**(1):44-51

[72] Neviaser AS, Hannafin JA. Adhesive capsulitis: A review of current treatment. The American Journal of Sports Medicine. 2010;**38**:2346-2356

[73] Schiefer M, Teixeira PF, Fontenelle C. Prevalence of hypothyroidism in patients with frozen shoulder. Journal of Shoulder and Elbow Surgery. 2017;**26**(1):49-55

[74] Li W, Lu N, Xu H, Wang H. Case control study of risk factors for frozen shoulder in China. International Journal of Rheumatic Diseases. 2015, Jun;**18**(5):508-513. DOI: 10.1111/1756-185X

[75] ISAKOS Upper Extremity Committee Consensus Statement. Shoulder Stiffness. Berlin: Springer-Verlag. 2014

[76] Zuckerman JD, Rokito A. Frozen shoulder: A consensus definition. Journal of Shoulder and Elbow Surgery, Elsevier. 2011;**20**(2):322-325

[77] Neviaser JS. Adhesive capsulitis and the stiff and painful shoulder. Orthopedic Clinics of North America. 1980;**11**:327-331

[78] Hand GC, Athanasou NA, Matthews T, Carr AJ. The pathology of frozen shoulder. Journal of Bone and Joint Surgery (British). 2007;**89**:928-932

[79] Bunker TD, Reilly J, Baird KS, Hamblen DL. Expression of growth factors, cytokines and matrix metalloproteinases in frozen shoulder. Journal of Bone and Joint Surgery (British). 2000;**82**:768-773

[80] Neviaser RJ, Neviaser TJ. The frozen shoulder: Diagnosis and management. Clinical Orthopaedics. 1987;**223**:59-64

[81] Warner JJP. Frozen shoulder: Diagnosis and management. Journal of the American Academy of Orthopaedic Surgeons. 1997;**5**(3):130-140

[82] Griegel-Morris P, Larson K, Mueller-Klaus K. Incidence of common postural abnormalities in the cervical, shoulder, and thoracic regions and their association with pain in two age groups of healthy subjects. Physical Therapy. 1992;**72**(6):425-431

[83] Urvoy P, Boileau G, Berger M, et al. Confrontation e validation de plusieurs methods d'evaluation des resultants après chirurgie de la coiffe des rotateurs. Revue de Chirurgie Orthopedique. 1991;**77**:171-178

[84] Beaton D, Richards RR. Assessing the reliability and responsiveness of five shoulder questionnaires. Journal of Shoulder and Elbow Surgery. 1998;**7**:565-572

[85] McKee MD, Yoo DJ. The effect of surgery for rotator cuff disease on general health status. Journal of Bone and Joint Surgery (American). 2000;**82**:970-979

[86] Brox JI, Staff PH, Ljunggren AE, Brevik JI. Arthroscopic surgery compared with supervised exercises in patients with rotator cuff disease (stage II impingement syndrome). BMJ. 1993;**307**:899-903

[87] Cho K, Song J, Lee H, Kim J, Rhee Y. The effect of subacromial bursa injection of hyaluronate in patients with adhesive capsulitis of shoulder joint: Multicenter, prospective study. Journal of Korean Academy of Rehabilitation Medicine. 2002;**26**:73-80

[88] Tamai K, Mashitori H, Ohno W, Hamada J, Sakai H, Saotome K. Synovial response to intraarticular injections of hyaluronate in frozen shoulder: A quantitative assessment with dynamic magnetic resonance imaging. Journal of Orthopaedic Science. 2004;**9**:230-234

[89] Tagliafico A, Serafini G, Sconfienza LM, et al. Ultrasound-guided viscosupplementation of subacromial space in elderly patients with cuff tear arthropathy using a high weight hyaluronic acid: Prospective open-label non-randomized trial. European Radiology. 2010;**21**:182-187

[90] Graff J, Richter KD, Pastor J. Effect of high energy shock waves on bony tissue. Urological Research. 1988;**16**:252-258

[91] Haupt G. Use of extracorporeal shock waves in the treatment of pseudarthrosis, tendinopathy and other orthopedic diseases. The Journal of Urology. 1997;**158**(1):4-11. DOI: 10.1097/00005392-199707000-00003

[92] Lohrer H, Nauck T, Vasileios Korakakis V, Malliaropoulos N. Historical ESWT paradigms are overcome: A narrative review. BioMed Research International. 2016;**2016**:7

[93] Chen YJ, Wang CJ, Yang KD, et al. Extracorporeal shock waves promote healing of collagenase-induced achilles tendinitis and increase TGF-beta1 and IGF-I expression. Journal of Orthopaedic Research. 2004;**22**(4):854-861

[94] Wang FS, Yang KD, Chen RF, Wang CJ, Sheen-Chen SM. Extracorporeal shock wave promotes growth and differentiation of bone-marrow stromal cells towards osteoprogenitors associated with induction of TGF-beta1. The Journal of Bone and Joint Surgery. 2002, Apr;**84**(3):457-461

[95] Wang FS, Wang CJ, Chen YJ, et al. Ras induction of superoxide activates ERK-dependent angiogenic transcription factor HIF-1alpha and VEGF-A expression in shock wave stimulated osteoblasts. Journal of Biological Chemistry. 2004;**279**:10331-10337

[96] Kearney CJ, Hsu HP, Spector M. The use of extracorporeal shock wavestimulated periosteal cells for orthotopic bone generation. Tissue Engineering. 2012, Jul;**18**:1500-1508

[97] Tamma R, dell'Endice S, Notarnicola A, Moretti L. Extracorporeal shock waves stimulate osteoblast activities. Ultrasound Med Biol. 2009, Dec;**35**(12):2093-2100

[98]   Wang CJ, Yang KD, Ko JY, Huang CC, Huang HY, Wang FS. The effects of shockwave on bone healing and systemic concentrations of nitric oxide (NO), TGF-b1, VEGF and BMP-2 in long bone non-unions. Nitric Oxide. 2009;20:298-303

[99]   Frairia R, Berta L. Biological effects of extracorporeal shock waves on fibroblasts. A Review. Muscle, Ligaments and Tendons Journal. 2011, Oct-Dec;1(4):138-147

[100] Saggini R, Di Stefano A, Saggini A, Bellomo RG. Clinical application of shock wave therapy in musculoskeletal disorders: Part I. Journal of Biological Regulators & Homeostatic Agents. 2015;29(3):533-545

[101] Saggini R, Buoso S, Pestelli G. Dolore E Riabilitazione. 1st ed. Minerva Medica, Torino, Italy. 2014

[102] Schmitz C, Császár N, Milz S. Efficacy and safety of extracorporeal shock wave therapy for orthopedic conditions: A systematic review on studies listed in the PEDro database. British Medical Bulletin. 2015;116:115-138. DOI: 10.1093/bmb/ldv047

[103] Mouzopoulos G, Stamatakos M, Mouzopoulos D, Tzurbakis M. Extracorporeal shock wave treatment for shoulder calcific tendonitis: A systematic review. Skeletal Radiology. 2007;36:803-811. DOI: 10.1007/s00256-007-0297-3

[104] Notarnicola A, Moretti B. The biological effects of extracorporeal shock wave therapy (ESWT) on tendon tissue. Muscles, Ligaments and Tendons Journal. 2012;2(1):33-37

[105] Vahdatpour B, Taheri P, Zade AZ, Moradian S. Efficacy of extracorporeal shock-wave therapy in frozen shoulder. International Journal of Preventive Medicine. 2014; 5(7):875-881

[106] Park C, Lee S, Yi CW, Lee K. The effects of extracorporeal shock wave therapy on frozen shoulder patients' pain and functions. Journal of Physical Therapy Science. 2015;27(12):3659-3661. DOI: 10.1589/jpts.27.3659

[107] Evans CH, Kraus VB, Setton LA. Progress in intra-articular therapy. Nature Reviews. Rheumatology. 2014;10(1):11-22. DOI: 10.1038/nrrheum.2013.159

[108] Gross C, Dhawan A, Harwood D. Glenohumeral joint injections. A review. Sports Health. 2013, Mar;5(2):153-159. DOI: 10.1177/1941738112459706

[109] Wittich CM, Ficalora RD, Mason TG, Beckman TJ. Musculoskeletal injection. Mayo Clinic Proceedings. 2009;84(9):831-837

[110] Song A, Higgins LD, Newman J, Jain NB. Glenohumeral corticosteroid injections in adhesive capsulitis: A systematic search and review. PM & R : The Journal of Injury, Function, and Rehabilitation. 2014;6(12):1143-1156

[111] Kim YS, Park JY, Lee CS, Lee SJ. Does hyaluronate injection work in shoulder disease in early stage? A multicenter, randomized, single blind and open comparative clinical study. Journal of Shoulder and Elbow Surgery. 2012;21:722-727

[112] Osti L, Berardocco M, di Giacomo V, Di Bernardo G, Oliva F, Berardi AC. Hyaluronic acid increases tendon derived cell viability and collagen type I expression in vitro: Comparative study of four different hyaluronic acid preparations by molecular weight. BMC Musculoskeletal Disorders. 2015;**16**:284

[113] Mathieu P, Conrozier T, Vignon E, Rozand Y, Rinaudo M. Rheologic behavior of osteoarthritic synovial fluid after addition of hyaluronic acid: A pilot study. Clinical Orthopaedics and Related Research. 2009;**467**(11):3002-3009. DOI: 10.1007/s11999-009-0867-x

[114] Speed CA. Fortnightly review: Corticosteroid injections in tendon lesions. BMJ. 2001;**323** (7309):382-386

[115] Saggini R, Di Stefano A, Capogrosso F, et al. Viscosupplementation with hyaluronic acid or polynucleotides: Results and hypothesis for condro-synchronization. Clinical Trials Journals. 2014;**4**:198. DOI: 10.4172/2167-0870.1000198

[116] Mitsui Y, Gotoh M, Nakama K, et al. Hyaluronic acid inhibits mRNA expression of proinflammatory cytokines and cyclooxygenase-2/prostaglandin E2 production via CD44 in interleukin-1-stimulated subacromial synovial fibroblasts from patients with rotator cuff disease. Journal of Orthopaedic Research. 2008;**26**(7):1032-1037

[117] Merolla G, Bianchi P, Porcellini G. Ultrasound-guided subacromial injections of sodium hyaluronate for the management of rotator cufftendinopathy: A prospective comparative study with rehabilitation therapy. Musculoskeletal Surgery. 2013;**1**:49-56

[118] Setuain I, Gonzalez-Izal M, Paularena A, Luque JL, Andersen LL, Izquierdo M. A protocol for a new methodological model for work-related shoulder complex injuries: From diagnosis to rehabilitation. BMC Musculoskeletal Disorders. 2017;**18**:70

[119] Michener LA, Walsworth MK, Burnet EN. Effectiveness of rehabilitation for patients with subacromial impingement syndrome: A systematic review. Journal of Hand Therapy. 2004;**17**:152-164

[120] Ashton-Miller JA, Wojtys EM, Huston LJ, Fry-Welch D. Can proprioception really be improved by exercises? Knee Surgery, Sports Traumatology, Arthroscopy. 2001;**9**: 128-136

[121] Reinold MM, Escamilla RF, Wilk KE. Current concepts in the scientific and clinical rationale behind exercises for glenohumeral and scapulothoracic musculature. The Journal of Orthopaedic and Sports Physical Therapy. 2009;**39**:105-117

[122] Myers JB, Oyama S. Sensorimotor training for shoulder injury: Literature review. Athletic Training and Sports Health Care. 2009;**1**:199-208

[123] Righetti GA, Magagni M, Marcolini G, Pari M, Galassi R. Trattamento propriocettivo nei pazienti operati di lesione della cuffia dei rotatori. European Journal of Physical and Rehabilitation Medicine. 2008;**44**:1

[124] Magagni GA, Righetti P, Mietti P, Marcolini M, Pari G, Galassi R. Nuovo sistema valutativo per la spalla. European Journal of Physical and Rehabilitation Medicine. 2008;**44**:1

3

Integral Management in Painful Shoulder Treatment: Anesthesiologist's Point of View

José Miguel Esparza Miñana

Abstract

Shoulder pain is a common complaint in clinical practice. The usual form of treatment is based on nonsteroidal anti-inflammatory drugs (NSAIDs), rest, rehabilitation and, as an alternative, a local injection into the joint. Due to the lack of oral medication and the lack of evidence, it is necessary to use different nonsurgical therapeutic alternatives. Pulsed radiofrequency produces a temporary nondestructive blockage being the most common technique in the management of shoulder pain. The application of pulsed radiofrequency on the suprascapular nerve has proven to be an effective method in the treatment of shoulder pain, with a decrease in pain that allows the rehabilitation of patients. The axillary or circumflex nerve provides motor innervation mainly to deltoids with branches to the teres minor, provides sensitive innervation to the lower, lateral, and anterior articular capsule, and innervates the humeral head and upper humeral neck. It has a cutaneous branch, which contributes sensitivity of the skin on the deltoids. Combined pulsed radiofrequency on the suprascapular nerve and on the circumflex nerve has been scarcely studied with very few references in the literature. The joint treatment by pulsed radiofrequency technique on suprascapular nerve and circumflex nerve can provide a complete and lasting relief of this pathology.

Keywords: shoulder, suprascapular nerve, circumflex nerve, radiofrequency, chronic pain

1. Introduction

Shoulder pain is a common problem with an estimated prevalence of 4–26%. It has been estimated that 20% of the general population will suffer shoulder pain throughout their life with a prevalence that can reach up to 50% [1]. This entity is responsible for approximately 16% of all musculoskeletal conditions only behind patients with low back pain.

The painful shoulder is the third most frequent reason for consultation of osteoarticular pathology, after low back pain and neck pain. Between 70 and 85% of the consultations are due to pathology of the rotator cuff [2]. In recent years, these conditions are increasing being a reason for increasing consultation in specialized services in the locomotor system. Although the rotator cuff and subacromial structures make up the majority of the presentations of painful pathology of the shoulder, we cannot forget other less frequent but not less important pain locations [3].

"Painful shoulder syndrome" is a frequent and debilitating disease of diverse etiologies and complex diagnosis, being more common in the female population, and especially after the 5th decade of life [4], in an age range between 45 and 65 years, although it can manifest itself in other age groups [5]. The prevalence increases with age, some professions, and certain sports activities.

Although most chronic shoulder problems can be treated conservatively with activity modification, oral medications, physical therapy, and possible injections of corticosteroids, there are cases where surgical intervention is required. Patients with continuous instability or disabling pain not responding to initial conservative measures may require prior surgical referral. Surgical or specialty referral should also be considered when the diagnosis is unknown [6].

Post-operative pain after shoulder surgery is severe in many patients. For many years, interscalene brachial plexus block has been the gold standard for controlling this pain. However, this is a blockage of the proximal brachial plexus, and therefore, is associated with extensive nerve block, resulting in significant side effects and possible complications.

2. Anatomy and biomechanics of the shoulder

The shoulder or shoulder girdle is the anatomical structure with greater mobility of the body, in turn is the most complex structure. The shoulder complex allows an arch of maximum mobility due to the multitude of structures involved in its stabilization: joints, ligaments, and muscles.

The articular complex of the shoulder is an enarthrosis, which confers an ample capacity of movement in the three axes and planes of the space, and this is due to the simultaneous and synchronous functioning of three joints: glenohumeral, acromioclavicular, and sternum-clavicular, in two sliding planes: scapulothoracic and subacromial deltoid. These joints intervene differently in the shoulder movements: in the first 90° of the abduction, the glenohumeral participates, between the 30 and the 135° the scalpulator is added, and from the 90° the acromioclavicular and the sternoclavicular are mobilized.

The glenohumeral joint consists of the head of the humerus and the glenoid cavity, has a large lax capsule, and is lined with a synovium, in which two muscles–tendinous systems of stabilization and fixation are joined. The humeral articular surface closes an ellipse, while the glenoid cavity offers a practically flat articular surface. The consequence of such mobility is the great instability of this joint, the joint being more frequently dislocated.

To compensate this instability, there are passive and active stabilizers. Within the passives is the joint capsule with anterior and posterior reinforcements that become independent in the upper and lower ligaments and the labrum. The labrum is a structure that surrounds the margin of the glenoid cavity conferring a greater congruence with respect to the humeral head. Among the active stabilizers, the most important elements are the components of the so-called rotator cuff.

The rotator cuff consists of the subscapularis muscle anteriorly, the supraspinatus and the long portion of the biceps above, and the infraespinatus and teres minor behind. Each of these muscles has its own rotating function (**Table 1**), but its joint action is the one that coapts the head of the humerus against the glenoid cavity and allows the elevation of the limb by the action of the deltoid [7].

	Muscle tendon	**Movements**
Upper region	Supraspinatus	Abduction
Posterior region	Infraspinatus, teres minor	External rotation
Anterior region	Subescapularis	Internal rotation
	Bicipital	Elbow flexion-supinatium

Table 1. Muscles and function.

3. Innervation of the joint

Sensory innervation of the shoulder joint is complex and involves contributions of the axillary, suprascapular, subscapular, musculocutaneous, and lateral pectoral nerves. Of these, the axillary and suprascapular nerves are considered the most important. However, variations and communications between the nerves are common.

It is important to have an exhaustive knowledge of the brachial plexus (**Figure 1**), since before considering a regional technique it is necessary to know well the innervation of the shoulder. The brachial plexus is formed by the anterior or ventral branches of the last four cervical spinal nerves: C5–C8 and the first thoracic: T1. These spinal nerves join together to form the primary trunks: upper (C5–C6), middle (C7), and lower (C8–T1). Just below the clavicle, the six divisions of the trunks will be formed, since each trunk is divided into anterior and posterior branches. From this moment, they are called secondary trunks or cords, which descend to the armpit. The axilla are denominated according to their relation with the axillary artery: anteroexternal (formed by the union of the upper and middle trunks), anterointernal (formed by the anterior branch of the inferior trunk), and posterior, formed by the posterior divisions of the primary trunks. Finally, each secondary trunk will give origin to the different terminal nerves: the posterior cord originates the axillary and radial nerves, the medial cord the ulnar nerve, and the lateral cord will give rise to the musculocutaneous nerve.

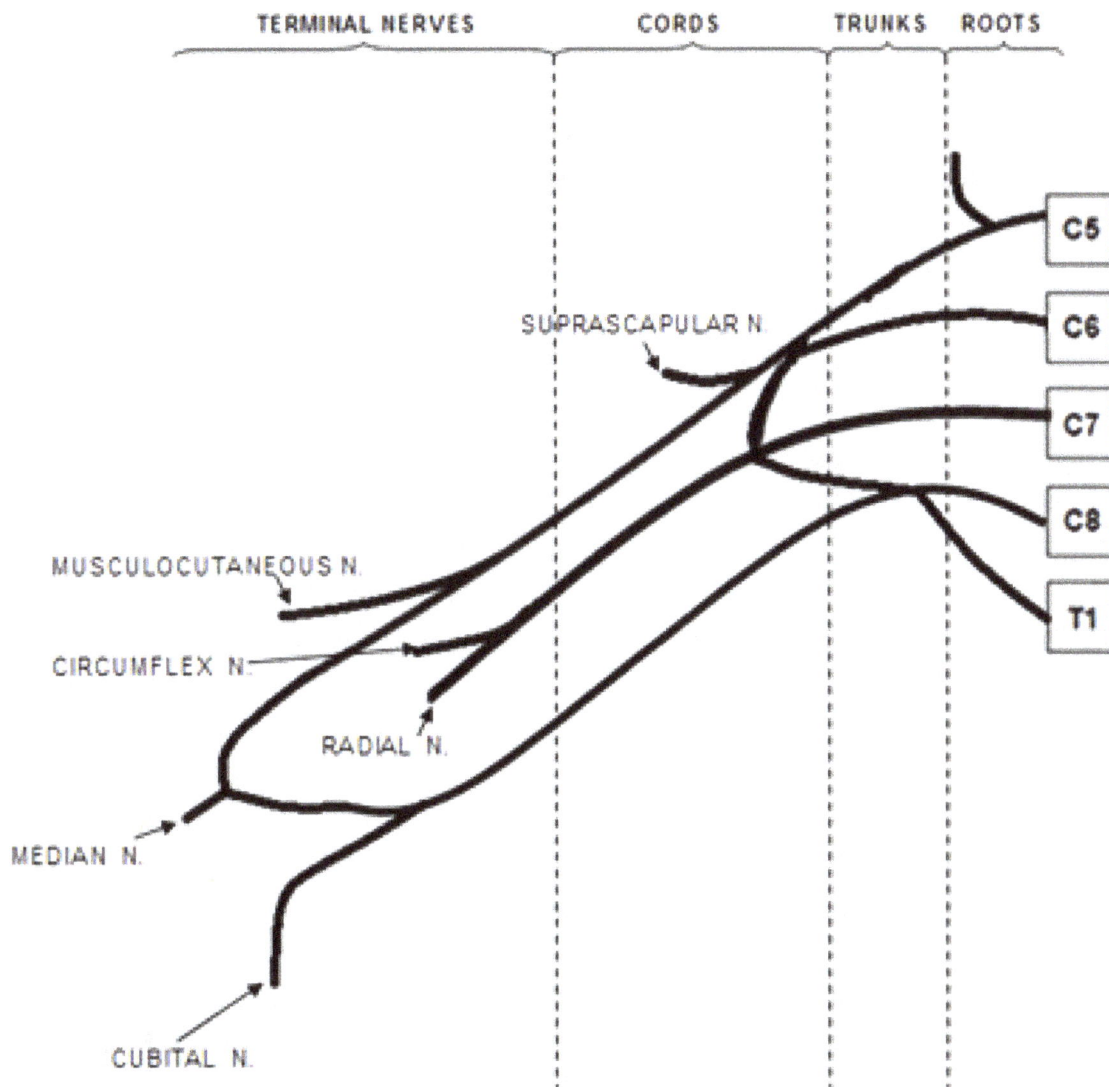

Figure 1. Division of the brachial plexus into its terminal branches.

The axillary plexus is responsible for both internal and cutaneous innervation of the shoulder, except for the upper part of the shoulder, which is innervated by the supraclavicular nerve originated in the lower part of the superficial cervical plexus (C3–C4). The articular innervation and the structures that surround it are mainly in charge of the axillary nerve or circumflex and the suprascapular nerve. To a lesser extent, they can be innervated by the musculocutaneous and subscapular nerve.

The suprascapular nerve is a mixed, motor and sensory nerve, formed by the direct union of the upper primary trunk of C5 and C6, with occasional contributions of C4 in some variants. It occurs laterally below the trapezius and omohyoid, and enters the supraspinatus fossa. The transverse scapular ligament closes the fossa on the nerve. In the suprascapular fossa, the nerve sends motor branches to the supraspinatus and infraspinatus muscles and some to the teres minor. It provides sensitive branches to the posterior glenohumeral capsule, acromioclavicular joint, and the coracohumeral ligament. In 15% of patients, the suprascapular nerve receives cutaneous sensory fibers from the upper side of the arm (deltoid) [8].

The axillary or circumflex nerve is a branch of the posterior secondary trunk (C5–C6). It forms on the lateral border of the subscapularis muscle, and is directed toward the posterior part of the surgical neck of the humerus. It runs below the shoulder joint about 2–3 mm below the lower capsule. Along with the posterior humeral circumflex artery, the nerve passes through a quadrilateral space forming a small aperture delimited by teres minor, teres major below, long head of medial biceps, and proximal humerus laterally. It provides motor innervation mainly to deltoids with branches to the teres minor, provides sensitive innervation to the lower, lateral, and anterior joint capsule, and innervates the humeral head and upper humeral neck. It has a cutaneous branch, which contributes sensitivity of the skin on the deltoids.

4. Intraoperative analgesic techniques

Multiple advantages present loco-regional anesthesia:

1. They allow a better control of the pain, decreasing the need for opiates, both intra- and post-operatively.

2. Decreases the incidence of nausea and vomiting, which increases patient satisfaction and decreases the average stay.

3. It provides an adequate muscular relaxation for the correct position of the patient.

4. Reduces intraoperative bleeding and promotes hemodynamic stability.

The reference technique for intraoperative analgesia is brachial plexus block at interscalene level [9]. Multiple approaches have been described: Winnie, Pippa, and Meier are the best known. Until not many years ago, the use of the neurostimulator for the accomplishment of the blockade was the gold standard technique. It was recommended to obtain a good response of the triceps (C5–C6) rather than a response of the biceps (C4–C5), ensuring a better distribution of the anesthetic.

With the development of ultrasound techniques and their progressive introduction into anesthesiology services, the use of neurostimulation for nerve localization in analgesic or anesthetic blocks has become obsolete. At the moment, the realization of a blockade that is not guided by ultrasound is not conceived.

The use of this technology brings a number of advantages. One of the most important is to be able to confirm the distribution of the local anesthetic around the nerve by direct vision. The use of ultrasound also improves safety, since we observe at all times the trajectory of the needle and its relation with neighboring structures (vascular, pleura, and solid organs). Another notable advantage is that the volume of local anesthetic is considerably lower. The correct extension of the anesthetic around the nerve allows a shortening of the latency of the blockade and a longer duration of the effect.

Brachial plexus block at interscalene level has been well described and widely used (**Figure 2**). The lack of impact of suprascapular nerve block on respiratory function makes it a good

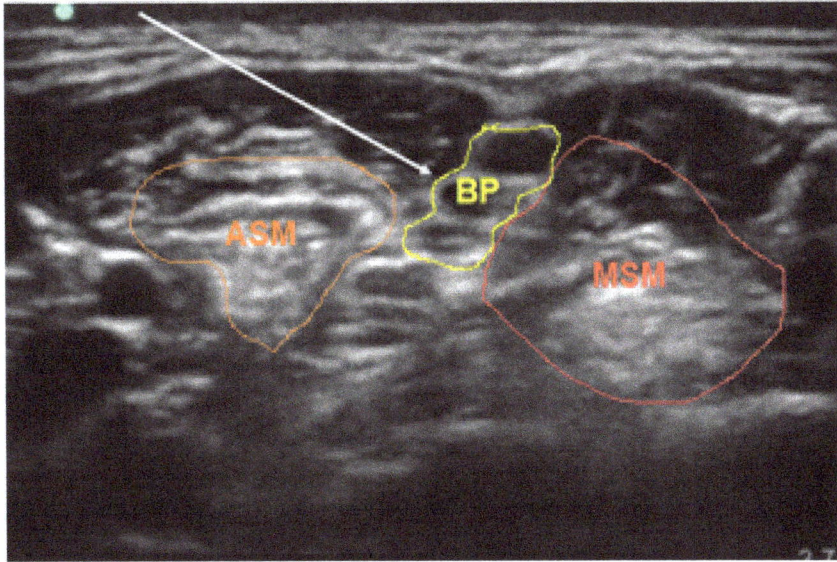

Figure 2. Ultrasound view of brachial plexus block at interscalene level. ASM, anterior scalene muscle; MSM, medium scalene muscle; BP, brachial plexus.

alternative in certain groups. To date, there have been no extensive trials comparing the efficacy and safety of the two, which could cause some reluctance to adopt suprascapular blockade as the regional technique of choice for shoulder surgery [10].

Good studies have recently appeared in this line. Dhir et al. [11] carried out a study with 60 patients in which they analyzed the combined blockade of the suprascapular and axillary nerves, comparing it with the interscalene brachial plexus block. They observed that the combined block provides nonequivalent analgesia compared to interscalene block in arthroscopic shoulder surgery. They conclude that while combined blockade provides better quality pain relief at rest and fewer adverse effects at 24 hours, interscalene block provides better postoperative analgesia. Therefore, for arthroscopic shoulder surgery, combined blockade may be a clinically acceptable analgesic option with a different analgesic profile compared to interscalene blockade.

However, Wiegel et al. [12] in a very recent study with 329 patients comparing the combined blockade of the suprascapular and axillary nerve with the interscalene blockade as analgesic techniques in arthroscopic shoulder surgery concluded that for outpatients subjected to arthroscopic surgery under general anesthesia, combined blockade seems preferable to interscalene. It provides excellent postoperative analgesia without exposing patients to alterations in mobility and the risks of interscalene blockade.

5. Postoperative analgesic techniques

In the immediate postoperative period, the patients present a very intense pain during the first hours. It is necessary to apply analgesic guidelines to control it, such as the combination of nonsteroidal anti-inflammatory drugs and intravenous opioids.

The use of catheters with continuous perfusion of local anesthetics accompanied by the possibility of self-administered boluses in shoulder surgery reduces the total dose of local anesthetic and the risk of side effects, and improves overall patient satisfaction. The use of an interscalene catheter is indicated mainly in patients who are going to undergo aggressive surgery with painful postoperative in the first 6 hours and in those patients who present the need for early and energetic rehabilitation. According to the type of surgery and patient characteristics, the catheter will be used between 3 and 5 days.

6. Analgesic techniques in treatment of chronic pain

The term "painful shoulder" encompasses all processes that determine pain in the anatomical region of the shoulder. "Painful shoulder syndrome" is a frequent and incapacitating pathology of diverse etiology and complex diagnosis. The causes of painful shoulder are multiple (**Table 2**). We should always ask if we are facing a disease of the shoulder or if it is a pain referred from another location.

Periarticular

   Rotator cuff tendinitis

   Rupture of the rotator cuff tendon

   Bicipital tendinitis

   Long biceps tendon rupture

Articular

   Frozen shoulder (adhesive capsulitis)

   Inflammatory arthritis

   Microcrystalline arthritis

   Dislocation, subluxation

Extrinsic causes

   Vascular or somatic origin

      Pancoast tumor, pneumothorax

      Aortic dissection, ischemic heart disease

      Atherosclerosis, vasculitis, aneurysms

   Neurological origin

      Spinal cord injury, peripheral nerve entrapment

      Fibromyalgia

      Complex regional pain syndrome

Table 2. Etiology of painful shoulder.

The most common symptom in the shoulder is pain. The patient's age, nature, and evolution of pain often lead to diagnosis. It is important to observe its onset, periodicity, location, character, irradiation, concomitant symptoms, and factors that aggravate or alleviate it. The radicular pain that radiates from the cervical region of the shoulder is almost always lacerating; on the other hand, the pain of tendinitis is diffuse, deaf, and continuous.

Subacromial syndrome (SAS), associated or not with rotator cuff tears, is a common cause of shoulder pain, especially in manual workers and athletes involving throwing. The most frequent clinical manifestation of this pathology is through a painful arch pattern between 90 and 120° of abduction. However, SAS can also be presented by a capsular pattern, appearing as a rigid shoulder, or with a pseudoparalytic pattern, in which the main manifestation is impotence for shoulder elevation. This pattern indicates a massive lesion of the rotator cuff with alteration of the kinematic pattern of the shoulder. Finally, a mixed pattern may appear in which several forms of presentation are manifested associated with each other [13].

There is a wide range of painful shoulder treatments beginning with conservative treatment, physical therapies with rest, thermal, physiotherapeutic exercises, drug treatment with nonsteroidal anti-inflammatory drugs (NSAIDs) or analgesics, and joint blockages. Radiofrequency techniques are proposed as a therapeutic alternative in cases refractory to the treatments described.

We have several therapeutic options. Conservative treatment is the first step among the different nonpharmacological alternatives. Modifying daily activity is a simple treatment to decrease shoulder pain. Specific recommendations based on avoiding or decreasing painful activity are the basis of treatment in rotator cuff pathology, glenohumeral joint arthritis, and adhesive capsulitis. Avoiding movement above the head eludes the painful arch between 60 and 120° [6]. There are therapeutic modalities designed to relieve pain directly: cold and heat, ultrasound, iontophoresis, as well as stretching and strengthening [14] exercises that aim to improve overall shoulder function.

In a systematic review, Camarinos et al. concluded that the benefit of nonpharmacological interventions is based on improving mobility, although improvement in function and quality of life is questionable. Fortunately, we also have a broad pharmacological array, although few medications are specifically approved for the treatment of chronic shoulder pain. Most of these are indicated only for bursitis [15]. Nonsteroidal anti-inflammatory drugs (NSAIDs) may be effective in 50–67% of patients, but have only been evaluated in short periods of time. There are no randomized studies comparing the effectiveness of NSAIDs with other analgesics or with a more conservative approach.

Due to the lack of oral medication and the lack of existing evidence, it is necessary to use different nonsurgical therapeutic alternatives [16]. Among the invasive techniques, intra-articular infiltration is a relatively simple technique that can provide adequate pain control. Intra-articular injection of corticosteroids provides better pain relief than oral NSAIDs in the short term.

A recent Cochrane [15] review comparing intra-articular injection with other nonphysiotherapeutic treatment interventions and including a multiple outcome study evaluated at many time points shows that intra-articular corticosteroid injection is significantly more beneficial than a combined physiotherapeutic approach (mobilization, exercise, and electrotherapy) in improving the main complaint at 3, 7, and 13 weeks, but not later. This benefit was maintained when combined with a second study that evaluated short-term pain and did not demonstrate significant differences between groups.

Several studies have evaluated the use of hyaluronic acid in the treatment of shoulder pain. The study by Abellán et al. [13] compared the treatment with subacromial infiltrations with hyaluronic acid and those of corticosteroids, considered as the gold standard, in the treatment of conservative treatment resistant shoulder pain. The results show that subacromial infiltration of hyaluronic acid decreases pain and improves joint function in the same way as corticosteroids. Corticosteroids improve the patients faster, while with hyaluronic acid the improvement is progressive, presenting the same results at 6 months.

Infiltrations would be indicated in the case of poor recovery 4–8 weeks after conservative treatment and in patients with severe pain limiting rehabilitation treatment. The following are the most frequent infiltration techniques:

6.1. Intra-articular infiltration

With corticosteroids, local anesthetic, NSAIDs or combined, it is not recommended to make more than three infiltrations.

1. Infiltration of the acromioclavicular joint: with the patient seated and the upper limbs resting on their thighs, the physician should be placed in front, in an anterior position and lateral to the shoulder to infiltrate. To identify the joint, it is useful to palpate the lateral epiphysis of the clavicle in the medial-lateral direction to locate a small depression usually painful under pressure. Injection can be done by superior or anterior approach.

2. Infiltration of the glenohumeral joint: it can be approached by posterior or anterior route, in the latter the anatomical relations are more important. With the patient seated and the upper limbs resting on their thighs we will position laterally to the shoulder to infiltrate, and placed in a plane anterior or posterior to the shoulder according to the way of approach. The posterior route is the safest route and the least technical complication.

3. Infiltration of the subacromial space: it is an efficient and economic technique, which has a double function, on the one hand, clinical confirmation of the diagnosis in the pathology of the rotator cuff and the subacromial syndrome and, on the other hand, its symptomatic treatment in both processes. There are several introduction windows in the subacromial space, but the most recommended and used in the clinic are the following two (**Figure 3**):

a. *Lateral path*: The puncture window is located in the space between the acromion and the humeral head, on the lateral side of the shoulder. The patient is placed with the shoulder in neutral position, with the elbow in 90° flexion and the hand on the thigh of the same side.

b. *Posterior path*: The puncture window is located just below the acromion on the posterior side of the shoulder. With the patient in the same anterior position, we placed behind this and located the posterolateral edge of the acromion, marking the point of infiltration just below it.

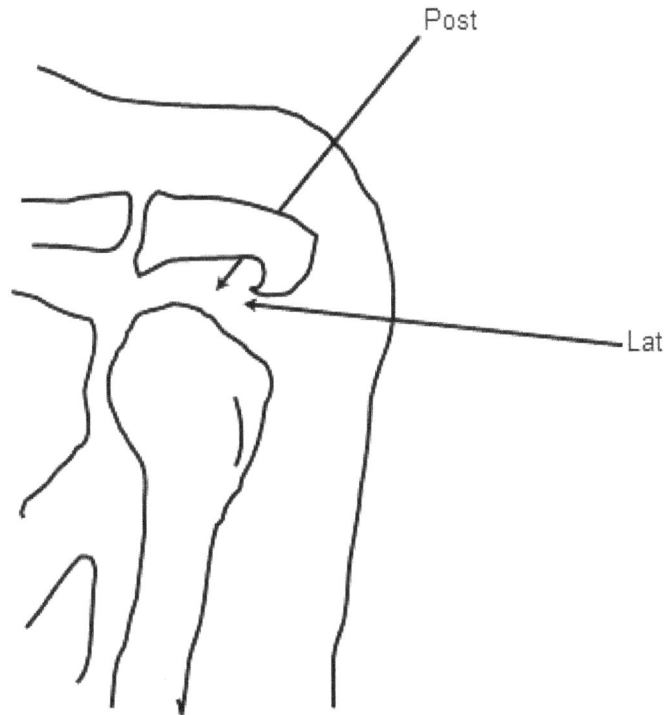

Figure 3. Infiltration of the subacromial space.

6.2. Suprascapular nerve block

Suprascapular nerve block appears to be effective in the treatment of chronic shoulder pain secondary to degenerative diseases and inflammatory diseases using injections of local anesthetic and corticosteroids. It also allows an early rehabilitation with adequate range of movements after reconstruction of shoulder or joint prosthesis. The development of ultrasound and the availability of echographs in the pain units have made it possible to use this technology to perform the blockade in a quick, simple, and practically free of complications.

In order to perform this ultrasound-guided block, we place the patient in a sitting or lateral position with the affected shoulder above. We will use a linear high frequency transducer (6–13 MHz). We performed an initial scan in sagittal orientation at the medial border of the scapula to identify the pleura. Later, we scan laterally with this orientation and move the transducer to visualize the spine of the scapula. If we move it cephalically, we will find the suprascapular fossa. If we move the transducer laterally, maintaining a transverse orientation, to identify the supraspinatus muscle and the suprascapular fossa, we will find the nerve as a round, hyperechoic image below the transverse scapular ligament in the scapular notch (**Figure 4**).

6.3. Axillary nerve block

As we have discussed at the beginning of the chapter, this nerve provides motor innervation mainly to deltoids and teres minor, provides sensitive innervation to the lower, lateral, and

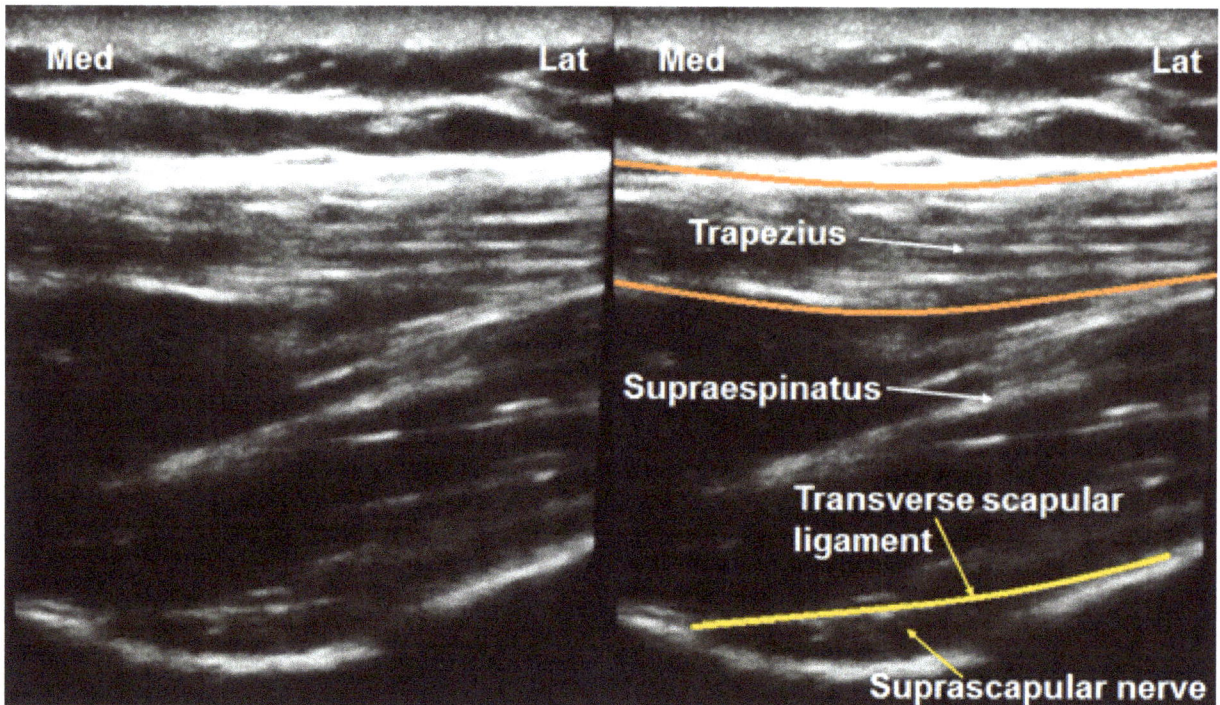

Figure 4. Ultrasound view suprascapular nerve.

anterior joint capsule, and innervates the humeral head and upper humeral neck. It has a cutaneous branch, which contributes sensitivity of the skin on the deltoids. To achieve more complete analgesic control of the shoulder joint, including the anterior region, we can perform a combined treatment of the suprascapular nerve and the axillary nerve. Therefore, axillary nerve block is performed as a complement to suprascapular nerve block to improve analgesic quality.

In order to perform this ultrasound-guided block, we place the patient in a sitting or lateral position with the affected shoulder above. We will use a linear high frequency transducer (6–13 MHz). We performed an initial scan at the posterior border of the arm at the deltoid level and identified the humeral head and the deltoid muscle. Between both the axillary nerves appear as a rounded and hyperechoic image (**Figure 5**).

6.4. Radiofrequency techniques

Radiofrequency was first used in the early 1950s. Cosman and Cosman [17, 18] described the use of high frequency currents (in the radiofrequency range) to produce lesions. A few years later, Sweet and Wepsic [19] made a second breakthrough in this field when he developed the first temperature-controlled radiofrequency system to produce lesions for the treatment of trigeminal neuralgia.

Currently, the use of electric currents by radiofrequency is a widely used clinical technique in the field of chronic pain treatment. It is a minimally invasive, percutaneous access technique in most cases, consisting of the application of a radiofrequency electric field (around 500 kHz)

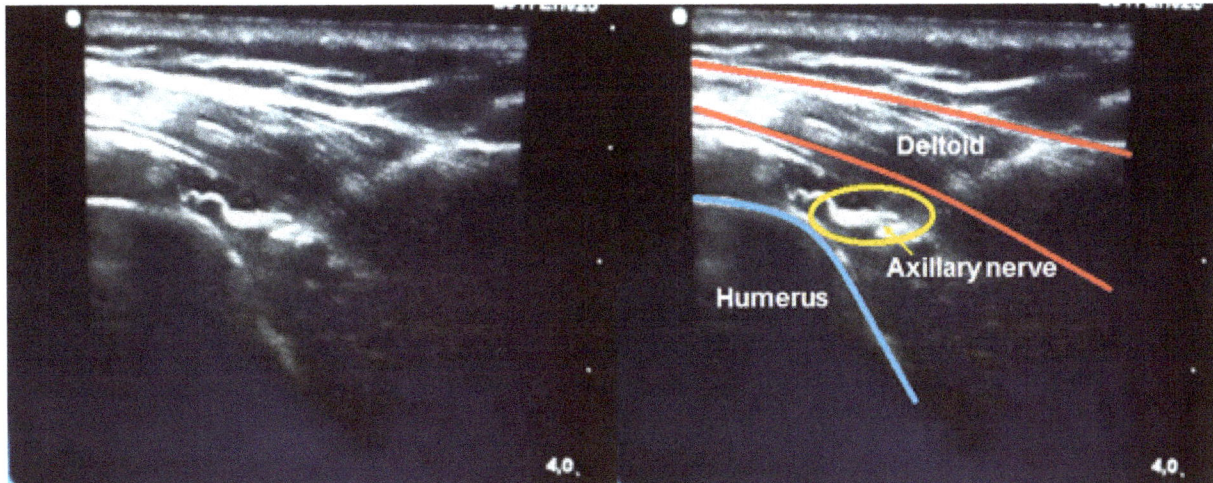

Figure 5. Ultrasound view axillary nerve.

around a tissue, through an applicator, that produces a modification in the treated target tissue, and consequently an alteration in the transmission of the painful stimulus.

The pulsed radiofrequency method (RFp) was initially used by Sluijter et al. [20]. To date, it has been used for the treatment of peripheral nerves and the dorsal root ganglion. It has been commonly applied for the treatment of low back pain, neck pain, and neuropathies with very good results. An advantage of RFp over conventional radiofrequency (RF) is that it generates very little discomfort and can be performed with very little or no pain on the patient while the technique is being performed.

The application of pulsed radiofrequency on the suprascapular nerve has proven to be an effective method in the treatment of shoulder pain, with a decrease in pain that allows the rehabilitation of patients [21]. On the other hand, it prevents repetitive infiltrations with local anesthetics and corticosteroids, which are not without undesirable effects [8, 22]. In order to achieve more complete analgesic control of the shoulder joint, including the anterior region, we can perform a combined treatment of the suprascapular nerve and the circumflex nerve.

In an observational study involving 16 patients with painful shoulder (13 patients with rheumatoid arthritis and 3 with osteoarthritis) and limited active movement of the joint, a combined block of the suprascapular nerve and the articular branches of the circumflex were performed. A mean reduction in pain intensity of 69% was observed with an improvement in ranges of motion (abduction, adduction, and flexion) that increased from 36 to 67% over a 13-week follow-up period [23].

The combined pulsed radiofrequency on the suprascapular nerve and on the axillary or circumflex nerve has been scarcely studied with very few references in the literature. Since the innervation of the shoulder joint is largely collected by these two nerves, the treatment by pulsed radiofrequency technique on suprascapular nerve and axillary or circumflex nerve can provide a complete and lasting relief of this pathology. In any case, more well-designed studies are needed to define the role of the combined technique in the treatment of the painful shoulder.

Author details

José Miguel Esparza Miñana

Address all correspondence to: miespmi@gmail.com

Escuela de Doctorado, Universidad Católica de Valencia San Vicente Mártir, Hospital de Manises, Valencia, Spain

References

[1] Esparza Miñana JM, Londoño Parra M, Villanueva Pérez VL, De Andrés Ibáñez J. Nuevas alternativas en el tratamiento del síndrome de hombro Doloroso. Semergen. 2012;38(1):40-43

[2] Dias D, Matos M, Daltro C, Guimarães A. Clinical and functional profile of patients with the painful shoulder syndrome (PSS). Ortopedia Traumatologia Rehabilitacja. 2008;10:547-553

[3] Benítez Pareja D, Trinidad Martín-Arroyo JM, Benítez Pareja P, Torres Morera LM. Estudio e intervencionismo ecoguiado de la articulación del hombro. Revista de la Sociedad Española del Dolor. 2012;19(5):264-272

[4] Camarinos J, Marinko L. Effectiveness of manual physical therapy for painful shoulder conditions: A systematic review. Journal of Manual and Manipulative Therapy. 2009;17:206-215

[5] Van der Windt DA, Koes BW, De Jong BA, Bouter LM. Shoulder disorders in general practice: Incidence, patient characteristics, and management. Annals of Rheumatic Diseases. 1995;5(4):959-964

[6] Burbank KM, Stevenson JH, Czarnecki GR, Forfman J. Chronic shoulder pain: Part II. Treatment. American Family Physician. 2008;77:493-497

[7] Basora M, Colomina MJ. Anestesia en Cirugía Ortopédica y en Traumatología. Capítulo: Hombro. Médica Panamericana; 2011. pp. 141-149

[8] Van Zundert J, de Louw A, Joosten E, Kesseles AG, Honig W, Federen PJ, et al. Pulsed and continuous radiofrequency current adjacent to the cervical dorsal root ganglion of the rat induces late cellular activity in the dorsal horn. Anaesthesiology. 2005;102:125-131

[9] Singelyn FJ, Lhotel L, Fabre B. Pain relief after arthroscopy shoulder surgery: A comparison of intraarticular analgesia, suprascapular nerve block and interscalene brachial plexus bloc. Anesthesia and Analgesia. 2004;99:589-592

[10] Heron M, Dattani R, Smith R. Interscalene vs suprascapular nerve block for shoulder surgery. British Journal of Hospital Medicine. August 2016;77(8):494-494

[11] Dhir S, Sondekoppam RV, Sharma R, Ganapathy S, Athwal GS. A comparison of combined suprascapular and axillary nerve blocks to interscalene nerve block for analgesia in arthroscopic shoulder surgery: An equivalence study. Regional Anesthesia and Pain Medicine. 2016 Sep–Oct;**41**(5):564-571. DOI: 10.1097/AAP.0000000000000436

[12] Wiegel M, Moriggl B, Schwarzkopf P, Petroff D, Reske AW. Anterior suprascapular nerve block versus interscalene brachial plexus block for shoulder surgery in the outpatient setting: A randomized controlled patient- and assessor-blinded trial. Regional Anesthesia and Pain Medicine. 2016 Sep–Oct;**41**(5):564-571. DOI: 10.1097/AAP.0000000000000436

[13] Abellán JF, Gimenez D, Melendreras E, Ruiz Merino G, Moreno MA. Treatment of persistent shoulder pain with subacromial sodium hyaluronate injection. Archivos de Medicina del Deporte. 2010;**XXVII**(140):449-456

[14] Vaquer L, Blasco L, Gozálvez E, Bayona MJ, Villanueva V, Asensio J, et al. Iontoforesis en el abordaje del paciente con dolor crónico. Revista de la Sociedad Española del Dolor. 2009;**16**:2758

[15] Green S, Buchbinder R, Hetrick S. Intervenciones fisioterapéuticas para el dolor del hombro. The Cochrane Library. 2008;Tomo **1**(2):65-75

[16] Andrews JR. Diagnosis and treatment of chronic painful shoulder: Review of non-surgical interventions. Arthroscopy: Journal of Arthroscopic and Related Surgery. 2005;**21**:333-347

[17] Cosman BJ, Cosman EC. Guide to Radiofrequency Lesion Generation in Neurosurgery. Radionics Procedure Technique Series Monographs. Burlington, MA: Radionics; 1974

[18] Cosman ER, Cosman BJ. Methods of making nervous system lesions. In: Wilkins RH, Ren-gachary SS, editors. Neurosurgery. Vol. 1. New York: McGraw-Hill; 1984. pp. 2490-2498

[19] Sweet WH, Wepsic JG. Controlled thermocoagulation of trigeminal ganglion and rootlets for differential destruction of pain fibers: I. Trigeminal neuralgia. Journal of Neurosurgery. 1974;**39**:143-156

[20] Sluijter ME, Cosman ER, Rittman WJ, Kleef M. The effects of pulsed radiofrequency fields applied to the dorsal root ganglion—A preliminary report. Pain Clinic. 1998;**11**(2):109-118

[21] Po-Chou, Kang L, Cheng-Loong. Pulsed radiofrequency lesioning of the suprascapular nerve for chronic shoulder pain: A preliminary report. Pain Medicine. 2009:**10**(1):70-75

[22] Haguichi Y, Nashold BS, Sluijter M, Cosman E, Pearlstein RD. Exposure of the dorsal root ganglion in rats to pulsed radiofrequency currents activates dorsal horn lamina I and II neurons. Neurosurgery. 2002;**50**:850-855

[23] Lewis RN. The use of combined suprascapular and circumflex (articular branches) nerve blocks in the management of chronic arthritis of the shoulder joint. European Journal of Anaesthesiology. 1999;**16**:37-41

4

Options Before Reverse Total Shoulder Replacement

Roger Hackney, Piotr Lesniewski and Paul Cowling

Abstract

Management of massive tears of the rotator cuff tears is one of the most difficult problems an upper limb surgeon encounters. Patients with similar tears can present with minimal discomfort through to a flail shoulder. There are a bewildering number of options available, many with published outcomes not always borne out in clinical practise. These range from rehabilitation, simple arthroscopic surgery, attempts at repair, complex tendon transfers and ultimately a reverse total shoulder replacement. More recently further options of patch augmentation and balloon arthroplasty have been added. This paper attempts to provide a critical assessment of the evidence available.

Keywords: massive rotator cuff tear, treatment options, repair, patch, augmentation, bridging

1. Introduction

Rotator cuff arthropathy has gained increased attention in recent years, partially because the ageing population has made it more prevalent. Cuff arthropathy is now one of the major problems a shoulder surgeon has to face nowadays in clinical practise. It is caused by a long-standing large or massive rotator cuff tear, leading to functional upriding of the humeral head due to unrestrained deltoid action and elevation of the effective centre of rotation of the gleno-humeral joint, often providing patients with a serious disability. The classic pseudoparalytic or flail shoulder with pain may be associated with degenerative changes in the gleno-humeral joint, but patients are frequently seen with minimal arthritic changes. The most definitive solution for treatment of rotator cuff arthropathy is the reverse Total Shoulder Arthroplasty (RTSA or RSA). Indications for RSA are mostly pain and to lesser extent loss of function. It often dramatically improves pain and function in patients with irreparable rotator cuff tears associated with pseudoparalysis. Satisfactory results can even be obtained in patients who have undergone previous procedures, such as rotator cuff repair [1]. Current available literature documents an implant survival rate of 91% at 10 years [2]. Given these promising results, it is no wonder that reverse total shoulder replacement is increasingly commonly used, making in 2015 over 45% of shoulder replacements performed in the UK according to the National Joint registry [3]. For patients with irreparable cuff tears aged 70 years or greater, it has practically replaced the other procedures. However successful, the longevity of reverse TSR does not yet match those expected for replacements of the hip and knee. For that reason, replacement before the age of 70 is not recommended by some authors [1, 3]. What are the options then for patients with symptomatic large and massive tears of the rotator cuff and little evidence of arthropathy, particularly in the younger patients unsuitable for reverse TSR?

In this chapter we will go through the most current concepts regarding massive and irreparable cuff tears, as well as cuff tear arthropathy. We will show the reader contemporary view on diagnosis and treatment of these conditions, but also share technique developed by the senior author and used in our daily practise.

2. Massive and irreparable rotator cuff tears

Massive rotator cuff tears (MRCT) make up to about 20% of all cuff tears [4, 5]. The number gets higher if we look at recurrent tears: in this group MRCT constitute of up to 80% [4, 5]. Cofield described cuff tear as a massive if its anteroposterior dimension reached or exceeded 5 cm [6]. Davidson and Burkhart in an attempt to add to their definition a second dimension, defined a massive tear as tears in which both coronal length and sagittal width were at least 2 cm long [7]. Gerber et al. defined a cuff tear as a massive once it involved a complete tear of at least two tendons [8]. Lädermann et al. advocated that to constitute a massive tear, at least one of two tendons should be involved, and should retract beyond the level of humeral head apex [9].

Once identified, massive tears can then be further classified by chronicity or with regard of a tear pattern.

If subdivided by the chronicity, tears can be defined as acute, acute on-chronic and chronic [10]. Acute MRCT are very infrequent, usually occurring after traumatic events and are more common among younger population [1, 10]. Individuals with a truly acute, traumatic massive cuff tear often present with a completely pseudoparalytic shoulder [1]. Plain radiographs should be taken to exclude a fracture and/or dislocation and may also document a wide joint space due to interposition of an avulsed cuff. MRI is used to assess the cuff, and in the presence of a massive tendon tear without the radiological signs of chronic tendon involvement (such as fatty muscle infiltration), earliest possible repair should be undertaken [1].

Apart from dramatic circumstances described above, most acute massive tears are actually acute on chronic tears where new onset or acutely deteriorating shoulder pain is due to underlying long lasting cuff pathology. These tears show often some signs of degeneration of the cuff and bony changes on greater tuberosity and acromion on radiograph [11].

Finally, the chronic massive tears are the most common and are found almost exclusively in older patients. They are associated with degenerative tendon changes such as myotendinous retraction, loss of musculotendinous elasticity, fatty infiltration of muscles, static (superior) subluxation of the humeral head, and ultimately, osteoarthritis [1].

If classified by anatomic tear pattern, MRTC usually fall into two distinct groups: posterosuperior and anterosuperior tears [12]. Most tears involve the supraspinatus and the infraspinatus, with or without the teres minor tendon, and these are considered as posterosuperior tears. Anterosuperior tears involve a complete tear of supraspinatus and subscapularis tendons [12]. Collin et al. made the tear pattern classification more precise and detailed, dividing the rotator cuff into five components: lower subscapularis, upper subscapularis, supraspinatus, infraspinatus and teres minor [13]. Depending on which component is involved in a tear, 5 tears patterns can be distinguished: Type A are supraspinatus and superior subscapularis tears; Type B are supraspinatus and entire subscapularis tears; Type C are supraspinatus, superior subscapularis, and infraspinatus tears; Type D, supraspinatus and infraspinatus tears; Type E are supraspinatus, infraspinatus, and teres minor tears [13]. This classification not only organizes all tears into tear pattern groups, but also aims at linking tear patterns with specific function loss. Therefore, Type A disruption typically causes a decrease in internal rotation strength with positive Belly press and Bear Hug tests, combined with a positive test for superior cuff insufficiency, e.g. empty can test. To a different extent the same is true for type B and C. Type D may show weakness of external rotation, while posterosuperior MRCT with an extension to the teres minor (Type E) may have an external rotation lag sign and often exhibit a positive Hornblower's sign (the inability to maintain external rotation with the arm abducted to 90) [13].

Fortunately irreparable rotator cuff tears (IRCT) are just a subgroup of massive tears, as some of the latter are amenable for repair. Exact incidence of IRCT is unknown, with some studies estimating it between 6.5% and 22.4% [10]. To be considered irreparable, a defect should be impossible to close at the time of surgery or show traits which have been empirically determined to be associated with structural failure of the repair [1]. According to Gerber, clinical signs which suggest that a repair is unlikely to be successful include:

- static anterosuperior subluxation with the head under the skin in front of the anterior acromion and associated pseudoparalysis of anterior elevation

- dynamic anterosuperior subluxation of the humerus upon resisted abduction

- positive lag sign and Hornblower's sign (both associated with substantial fatty infiltration of infraspinatus and teres minor respectively) [14, 15].

The imaging finding most commonly associated with irreparability of the cuff tear is a fatty infiltration of cuff muscle which equals or exceeds 50% of muscle's volume determined by CT or MRI (stages 3 and 4 of fatty infiltration according to Goutallier) [16]. Fatty degeneration is irreversible even with successful complete repair and leads to reduced function of the rotator cuff musculature [8, 17]. Some authors reported that in higher stages (Goutallier 3 and 4) of fatty infiltration, MRCT may fail to heal in up to 92% of cases. Another key imaging finding helping to predict irreparability of a tear is a static superior subluxation of a glenohumeral joint with an acromiohumeral interval of 7 mm or less. Also static anterior subluxation observed in CT scan or MRI appears to be indicative of irreparability of the tear [1].

3. Clinical signs and symptoms

As the incidence of rotator cuff tears increases with age, especially after age 60, elderly patients are the most likely group to seek help due to massive rotator cuff tears [10, 18]. Some of them might report a traumatic event and an acute loss of function, with or without previous symptoms; however, most will deny any noticeable trauma and complain of variable levels of pain [10]. It is important to ascertain that the pain reported by the patient is actually caused by the massive cuff tear, and not from another source.

If it is accompanied by stiffness, especially with limitation of passive external rotation and passive glenohumeral abduction, it is very likely that the pain is due to adhesive capsulitis rather than MRCT.

Acromioclavicular joint pain, though different from the usual rotator cuff pain [19] is the second most common cause of pain that is not caused by, but is occasionally [1] attributed to rotator cuff tear.

Loss of function and disability are the next biggest complaint, as MRCT is always accompanied by some degree of shoulder weakness. This weakness is especially marked with the limb away from patient's body. Anterosuperior tears usually result with painful weakness of elevation. Posterosuperior tears and global tears cause weakness of elevation and external rotation [20]. This usually spans from hardly any perceived weakness to so-called pseudoparalysis of elevation and/or external rotation [1]. Pseudoparalysis of anterior elevation describes the inability to elevate the arm to 90 deg. in the presence of unrestricted passive range of glenohumeral motion and in the absence of any neurologic impairment [21]. Pseudoparalysis of external rotation describes complete loss of active external rotation power in the presence of unrestricted passive external rotation and in the absence of neurologic impairment [1]. Collin et al. demonstrated that dysfunction of the entire subscapularis and supraspinatus or three rotator cuff muscles are risk factors for pseudoparalysis [13]. There are studies suggesting that primary arthroscopic repair can lead to reversal of preoperative pseudoparalysis in 90% of patients, but this number drops to 43% in revision surgeries [22].

Examination of the patient with suspected massive or irreparable rotator cuff tear should be performed with patient's torso exposed allowing proper comparison between two shoulders. Any atrophy in the supraspinatus or infraspinatus fossa should be noted, indicating a chronic tear. If the coracoacromial arch is incompetent, the outline of humeral head might be more prominent due to anterosuperior subluxation. Visible deltoid atrophy is especially of concern in patients with previous open surgeries. The long head of the biceps tendon might be affected by massive cuff tears and is often torn resulting in a 'Popeye' deformity (a visible bulge just proximal to the elbow).

Active and passive range of movement should of course be assessed and compared with the contralateral side. Active shoulder motion is usually decreased. Limitations of passive motion may be due to scar tissue formation associated with chronic tears, but these are usually mild and not very painful. It is important to discern this from the often much more painful adhesive capsulitis.

In patients with anterosuperior tears, significant weakness of the subscapularis will be noted. The bear hug test will most likely be positive. The belly-press manoeuvre, which tests the upper portion of the subscapularis muscle, is more likely to be abnormal than the lift-off test, which mainly reflects the lower subscapularis muscle function [10, 23]. Increased passive external rotation of the shoulder may also be present [10].

Two provocative manoeuvres can determine the extent of the posterosuperior cuff involvement. The external rotation lag sign. If the patient cannot actively maintain maximal external rotation of the shoulder with the elbow by his side, the test is considered positive for the infraspinatus tendon tear. The Hornblower's sign tests the integrity of teres minor [10]. With the elbow supported, the patient is asked to maintain maximal shoulder external rotation with the shoulder abducted to 90°. Inability to maintain this position is highly sensitive for teres minor tear [15]. The supraspinatus tendon tear is always involved and so patients from both these groups should show weakness of supraspinatus strength (positive empty can test).

4. Investigations

Plain radiographs are of a great value to the evaluation. They provide information on the glenohumeral joint, acromial morphology, and the position of the humeral head. Standard evaluation consists of anteroposterior, axillary, and an outlet or scapular Y views. Grashey view (a true anteroposterior view) is most helpful to show the status of the glenohumeral joint, whereas an outlet and scapular Y views can be useful to examine acromial pathology [10]. Plain anteroposterior views will demonstrate any upriding of the humeral head and any osteoarthritic changes. Decreased interval between the humeral head and undersurface of the acromion is often associated with massive and irreparable cuff tears. This distance, the acromiohumeral interval (AHI), measures 7–14 mm in healthy shoulders [24] and as previously mentioned if it falls below 7 mm, the probability of successful cuff repair drastically decreases [25]. Hamada et al. [26] demonstrated correlation between progression of rotator cuff tear and reduction of AHI. He developed a radiographic classification of massive rotator cuff tear arthritis which divides massive rotator cuff tears into 5 grades: in Hamada Grade 1 the AHI is maintained, and narrows in Grade 2. Acetabulization (concave deformity of the acromion undersurface) in addition to the Grade 2 narrowing is classified as Grade 3. In Grade 4, narrowing of the glenohumeral joint is added to the Grade 3 features, and Grade 5 comprises instances of humeral head collapse [26]. Walch et al. recognized a group with massive tears that demonstrated glenohumeral narrowing without acromial acetabulization. Thus, they divided Grade 4 of Hamada into two subtypes: Grade 4A, glenohumeral arthritis without subacromial arthritis (acetabulization); and Grade 4B, glenohumeral arthritis with subacromial arthritis (Grade 4 of Hamada et al.). These subtypes allowed for more specific classification of patients and almost all patients could be classified [26].

CT scan was the original investigation described by Goutallier in assessment of fatty atrophy, and can still be used for patients where any bony changes need to be more accurately determined and the state of muscle wasting and atrophy. Goutallier et al. classified muscle quality by the amount of fatty infiltration in the rotator cuff muscle as identified on CT in the axial plane, with a thorough analysis of the whole muscle belly [16]. They graded muscular fatty degeneration into 5 stages: Stage 0 is a normal muscle with no fatty infiltration and stage 1 is a muscle in which some fatty streaks can be seen on CT. Stage 2 is a muscle with substantial fatty atrophy but still affecting less than 50% of visible muscle. In stages 3 and 4 fatty atrophy affects 50% and over 50% of muscle respectively [16]. According to various authors fatty muscle infiltration beyond Goutallier stage 2 represents a non-functional muscle belly making a successful repair of its tendon virtually impossible [1, 16].

One of the most common imaging modalities for assessing the rotator cuff is magnetic resonance imaging (MRI). It can reliably identify and characterize the rotator cuff tendon tears [27]. MRI scan is easier to read in assessing the size of any rotator cuff tear and both muscle wasting and fatty atrophy, but patients with sore shoulders may struggle to stay still for the duration of the scan which may take 45 min. With the growing popularity of magnetic resonance imaging Goutallier classification was adapted to MRI. Some authors correlated it with surgical outcomes and retear rates [10] and found that like for CT the advanced degree of fatty infiltration (over 2 Goutallier) on preoperative MRI was a strong predictive factor of cuff repair failure [10].

It is worth remembering that for MRI, the Goutallier scoring uses a different plane compared to CT. It is no longer the axial plane but the most lateral parasagittal image on which the scapular spine is still in contact with the scapular body (Y view) [28]. This makes the method prone to false interpretation in cases of massive cuff tears, because severe muscle-tendon retraction can cause bunching of the muscle that may actually create an illusion of a larger muscle belly than in reality [10]. Some authors reported the use of so-called 'tangent sign' [29] as an indicator of advanced fatty infiltration [30] and as a predictor of whether a rotator cuff tear will be reparable [31]. A tangent sign is positive when atrophied supraspinatus muscle falls below a tangent line drawn between superior border of coracoid process and superior margin of scapular spine. This is assessed, just like Goutallier score, on the most lateral MRI image on which both coracoid process and scapular spine are still in contact with scapular body [32]. However a recent study by Kim et al. showed that tangent sign alone was not a good predictive indicator of outcome of massive cuff repair. According to authors the single most predictive factor of successful repair in MRCT remains infraspinatus fatty infiltration <3 according to Goutallier [32].

Another important diagnostic modality is a ultrasound scan, which has become a popular modality for evaluating rotator cuff pathology because of its low cost and reliability in identifying the presence of a tear and its size even during the postoperative period [10]. Unfortunately ultrasound cannot penetrate through bone and may not provide accurate information about large rotator cuff tears where the tendon edges have retracted medial to the lateral acromial border [33]. Its optimal use is also notoriously dependent on the technician's experience.

5. Treatment options

5.1. Conservative treatment

Conservative treatment is often appropriate if a tear is proven to be irreparable, or the patient does not want operative intervention. Patients without any significant symptoms of pain may benefit from the anterior and middle deltoid rehabilitation programme. This has a success rate of about 30% and is particularly useful for those patients with loss of function without a great deal of pain. In this group conservative treatment may lead to a very satisfactory clinical situation with restoration of active arm elevation but to an inevitable increase in joint degeneration [1]. Zingg et al. [34] have documented a surprisingly good clinical outcome using non-operative treatment with a substantial structural deterioration of cartilage, tendon, and muscle.

In general, in irreparable cuff tears non-operative management is attempted for 6 months before considering surgery [9]. Typical treatment includes physiotherapy, anti-inflammatory and analgesic drugs, re-education, acupuncture and judicious use of subacromial (which in case of MRCT are also intraarticular) injections. Injections of either corticosteroids or hyaluronic acid are used. While repeated intraarticular steroid injections are discouraged by some authors as being largely ineffective [35, 36], others pointed out on a good and comparable therapeutic effect of both dexamethasone and sodium hyaluronate [37]. Hyaluronans are meant to act by blocking pain receptors, stimulating endogenous hyaluronan production and have a direct anti-inflammatory effect by inhibiting leukocyte action [38]. These injections have been shown to be of benefit for early and late osteoarthritis of the shoulder [39, 40]. A series of infiltrations with hyaluronic acid (once a week for 3 weeks) followed by rehabilitative treatment yielded significant pain reduction, improvement of range of motion, and autonomy in daily life activities [41] in a cohort of 22 patients (mean age 78y) with rotator cuff tears.

Conservative treatment does not substantially alter the course of the natural history of massive tears and as such can only be advised for patients whose cuff tears are already irreparable and who for various reasons would not be suitable for operative treatment [1].

Somewhere in between conservative and surgical treatment is a place for supra scapular nerve block and ablation. This salvage procedure can be used for pain relief where this is the major symptom, after initial conservative therapies have been exhausted [42] and the patient is not fit for major surgery, or does not want an operation. The suprascapular nerve is derived from the upper trunk of the brachial plexus (C5, C6) and is a mixed motor and sensory nerve. It provides the main sensory innervation to the posterior shoulder joint capsule, acromioclavicular joint, subacromial bursa, coracoclavicular and coracohumeral ligament [43] and motor branches to both supra and infraspinatus muscles. Blockade of the suprascapular nerve has been shown to improve chronic pain in numerous studies [44]. Among different techniques described are supra scapular nerve blocks (SSNB) [42], percutaneous SSN pulsed radiofrequency and arthroscopic SSN neurectomy [45]. Pulsed radiofrequency (PRF) works by delivering an electrical field to neural tissue rather than thermal coagulation and affects the smaller pain fibres more than the larger motor fibres, thus preserving any residual motor function [45]. There is morphologic evidence that PRF is less neurodestructive than CRF (continuous radiofrequency) and it is possible that nerve fibres may regenerate after PRF treatment [42]. Kane et al. [42] showed that pulsed radiofrequency to the suprascapular nerve in a cohort of 12 patients with painful cuff tear arthropathy resulted in a significant improvement in Constant, Oxford and Visual Analogue scores at 3 months. In their technique suprascapular notch was identified by use of direct visualization with an image intensifier. The landmark to guide the initial entry point was a line drawn along the length of the scapular spine, bisected with a vertical line from the angle of the scapula. A radiofrequency needle was introduced through the skin, 2.5 cm along the line of the spine in the upper outer quadrant, and then guided to the edge of the suprascapular notch by use of the image intensifier. The nerve was located accurately by stimulating at 2 Hz (threshold <0.5 V). PRF was applied for 120 s 2 or 3 times. The total treatment time was 6–8 min.

Nizlan et al. [46] described an arthroscopic SSN neurectomy technique in patients who were poor surgical candidates for shoulder arthroplasty with significant chronic pain [45]. They performed arthroscopic examination through the standard posterior viewing portal first, confirming a complete and irreparable rotator cuff tear. A lateral working portal was created a few centimetres from the lateral edge of the acromion at the level of the posterior border of the acromioclavicular joint. Through this portal, a radiofrequency device and a shaver were used to clear the soft tissue within the spinoglenoid notch to identify the nerve at the floor of the notch. Once the nerve was identified on the floor of the spinoglenoid notch, it was traced proximally towards the transverse scapular ligament. The nerve was then divided proximally by use of the ablator at the suprascapular notch and distally at the floor of the spinoglenoid notch. They used their technique for severe shoulder pain treatment in a group of 20 patients 17 with a rotator cuff arthropathy, two with glenohumeral arthritis and one with a rotator cuff-deficient shoulder following an unsuccessful arthrodesis [46]. At an average follow-up of 29 months, 75% of their patients reported good to excellent pain relief scores.

5.2. Surgical treatment

5.2.1. Arthroscopic debridement with or without long head of the biceps tenotomy

Debridement of rotator cuff tears has been known to be associated with a satisfactory short term results, especially in patients with low demands [47–49]. The goal of the surgery is to remove the sources of pain; therefore, the torn edges of the rotator cuff tendons are debrided and a gentle bursectomy is completed. Complete anterior acromioplasty should be avoided in the setting of a massive tear as it may put coracoacromial ligament at risk and lead to postoperative anterosuperior subluxation of humeral head [50]. As it is reported that lateral acromion might be responsible for more impingement than the anterior part [51] some recommend lateral acromioplasty in addition to limited anterior acromioplasty [52, 53]. Despite these concerns, however, when Rockwood et al. [54] first proposed open debridement for treatment of massive cuff tears in 1995, he performed it with aggressive acromioplasty and complete release of the coracoacromial ligament. In this study, 50 patients (53 shoulders) where followed up at an average of 6.5 years, with 83% of patients having a satisfactory outcome with a significant decrease in pain. The average active elevation improved from an average 105° to 140° [54]. Gartsman et al. [55] reported positive outcomes with open debridement for patients with massive rotator cuff tendon tears, but noted a decrease in strength and suggested that this weakness may be due to the incompetent coracoacromial ligament and the loss of superior humeral head containment. He also showed that superior head migration or incompetent subscapularis or teres minor were a negative prognostic factors for this treatment [55].

If sole debridement and acromioplasty do not suffice, a tuberoplasty might be an alternative or a good addition to treatment [56]. Described by Fenlin et al. [57] in 2002, its main goal is to contour and reshape the greater tuberosity to create a smooth congruent articulation between the greater tuberosity of the humerus and the under surface of the acromion. An arthroscopic tuberoplasty technique was presented by Scheibel in 2004 and described as 'reversed arthroscopic subacromial decompression' [56]. Studies by Verhelst et al. and Lee et al. [58, 59] confirmed the benefits of the procedure as an option in patients with irreparable cuff tears, showing good and excellent results. Both authors highlighted importance of maintaining the coracoacromial arch as a passive stabilizer to anterior and superior subluxation of the proximal humerus.

The management of the long head of biceps (LHB) tendon at the time of debridement is still controversial. Tenotomy of the biceps was described as a routine pain treatment in rotator cuff disease by Walch et al. in 1997 [60]. Concerns about the safety of this treatment were expressed as according to some, the biceps tendon acts to depress the humeral head in absence of the rotator cuff tendons [61]. In theory, release of the long head of the biceps might lead to further proximal migration of the humeral head. However, a number of studies found no proof to support these concerns [47, 62] The available evidence suggests that the proximal long head of biceps tendon may be a source of significant pain and that LHB tenotomy provides a reasonable pain relief without the additional risk of superior migration of the humeral head. A couple of multicentre studies identified LHB tenotomy as a valuable option giving good pain relief in patients with MRCT [63, 64]. It seems also the results are the same whether it is tenotomy alone or with tenodesis [1].

In summary, it seems that debridement of rotator cuff tendon stumps with subacromial decompression leads to satisfactory clinical results with large majority of patients with MRCT. A tuberoplasty might also be considered in this patients group. Coraco-acromial ligament, a major restraint against superior migration of the humeral head, should be handled with care, and can be detached but should not be resected in this group of patients [65, 66]. A biceps tenotomy, with or without tenodesis seems to be a safe additional procedure, helping decreasing the pain associated with massive cuff tears [64]. Debridement gives good pain relief but does not influence the progression of joint degeneration, so its role should be limited to treatment of irreparable cuff tears in low-demand patients whose primary complaint is pain [1].

5.2.2. Rotator cuff repair

If a massive rotator cuff tear can successfully be repaired, short- and long-term clinical results are excellent and joint degeneration is halted or at least markedly decelerated [67, 68]. According to Burkhart the goal of a repair, even if partial, is to restore force couples acting on the joint [50]. During shoulder motion, the rotator cuff muscles act together to centralize the humeral head against the glenoid fossa and balance the force couples about the glenohumeral joint. A force couple is a pair of forces that act on an object and cause it to rotate. For the object to be in equilibrium, the forces must be balanced, so must be equal in magnitude and opposite in direction [50]. In the shoulder, Inmann et al. [50] described coronal plane force couple as a result of the balance of moments created by the deltoid versus those created by inferior cuff (infraspinatus, trees minor and subscapularis). In order to oppose the superior pull of deltoid exerted during abduction, the inferior cuff must be intact. The second important force couple is the transverse force couple where action of subscapularis anteriorly is balanced against the posterior cuff (infraspinatus and trees minor). In massive cuff tears extending far posteriorly, the weak posterior cuff is unable to balance the anterior moment created by subscapularis and the equilibrium in transverse plain is not maintained. If large enough and affecting the inferior part of the cuff, the massive tear can disrupt the equilibrium in coronal plane. Lack in balance in two planes will lead to anterior and superior translation of the humeral head and inability to maintain a stable fulcrum of motion [50]. So during the repair it is more important to balance these force couples in coronal and transverse planes, than just to cover cuff defect [50].

In the context of the irreparable rotator cuff tear, it was felt by Burkhart that even partial repair of these tears could lead to good outcomes provided that the balance in both planes was restored [69]. Another important concept introduced by this author, helping to understand cuff anatomy, mechanics and principles for repair was 'suspension bridge analogy'. When viewed arthroscopically the undersurface of the intact cuff shows a 'cable-like' thickening of the capsule, surrounding a thinner crescent of tissue that inserts into the greater tuberosity of the humerus [50]. This 'cable-like' structure is a thickening of the coracohumeral ligament and extends from its anterior attachment to the greater tuberosity just posterior to the long head of the biceps, to its posterior attachment near the inferior border of the infraspinatus. This cable potentially serves a protective role, transferring the stress along the rotator cable, thereby stress-shielding much thinner, avascular crescent tissue, thus the analogy to the suspension bridge. The cuff can still successfully serve its function as long as the cable is intact. This is how authors explained good results of even partial repair, without watertight closure, but with reconstruction of cable attachments [50].

Although very difficult, complete repair of the massive cuff tears is not impossible, but requires very gentle soft tissue handling. One of the most significant issues in repairing a massive rotator cuff tears is the ability to mobilize the retracted tendon back to its insertion [10]. All adhesions around the cuff tendons must be removed. Common locations for these adhesions include the undersurface of the acromion, the posterior deltoid, the bursa and the interval between the undersurface of the tendon and labrum or glenoid [10]. If these release do not give relatively tension-free repair, additional techniques must be used. Tauro popularized the arthroscopic technique of the interval slide, which Burkhart [10, 50] later redefining it as an anterior interval slide, adding that a posterior slide as an option. Anterior interval slide is performed by releasing the rotator interval between subscapularis and supraspinatus, exposing the coracoid process. In its later version, named 'anterior interval slide with continuity', the rotator interval is released medially to the so-called 'comma tissue'. This comma tissue, a remnant of the bicep pulley, connects the superior border of subscapularis tendon with the anterior edge of supraspinatus and helps to repair one of the tendons after the other has been repaired. The posterior interval slide is performed between the supraspinatus and infraspinatus tendons up to scapula spine [10, 50].

Another useful technique, helping to decrease the tension from the cuff tissue and thus making massive cuff tears repairable, is a margin convergence [50]. This technique converts irreparable U-shaped and L shaped defects into more a manageable crescent-shaped tears that can be repaired completely [50]. The tears are initially repaired with side-to-side suturing of anterior and posterior leaves of the tear, from medial to lateral. This causes the free margin of the cuff to converge laterally towards the bony bed of the greater tuberosity, and then the free margin can be securely anchored to the bone with relatively little strain [50].

To account for poor quality tissue (osteopenic tuberosities, weak and non-elastic tendons)in chronic tears, and to minimize the likelihood of a retear after the repair, various other techniques have been described. These include the use of stronger sutures, various suturing configurations (e.g. Mason-Allen technique), larger and more rigid suture anchors, and bone tunnels, with or without a metallic plates and buttons [70, 71].

If the complete repair is impossible, the previously mentioned partial repair seems to represent a reasonable option in this challenging subset of patients [45]. The main goal of partial repair is to achieve sufficient tendon healing to regain relatively pain-free overhead activity [50]. To accomplish this, the rotator cuff repair must satisfy 5 biomechanical criteria:

- force couples must be balanced in coronal and transverse planes;

- a stable fulcrum kinematic pattern must be re-established;

- the residual defect should occupy a minimal surface area; and

- the residual defeat must possess edge stability.

These five criteria can be achieved by balancing the force couples between the anterior and posterior portions of the shoulder, which requires an intact subscapularis muscle anteriorly, an intact inferior half of infraspinatus posteriorly and preferably intact attachments of the rotator cable [50]. Although shoulder strength may not improve after this intervention, function is usually enhanced because of relief from pain caused by mechanical impingement [9].

There is a lack of strong evidence showing that either arthroscopic or open rotator cuff repair is superior. If the repair heals by either approach, the results are comparable. Despite high structural failure rates of the tendon in massive rotator cuff repair (retear rates of 34–94% have been reported [1], clinical outcome scores remain consistently good when compared with preoperative values [1, 72].

5.2.3. Tendon transfers

For those patients whose rotator cuff tendon cannot be repaired completely or even partially to provide symptomatic relief, a salvage reconstruction with muscle-tendon transfer may be considered [73]. The ideal candidate for this type of procedure is a young, active patient with an irreparable rotator cuff tendon tear and minimal glenohumeral arthritis whose primary complaint is weakness [10]. Various tendons transfer techniques has been described for patients with massive irreparable tears, with the most common being latissimus dorsi with or without the teres major, pectoralis major, and trapezius [10, 41].

Pectoralis major transfer is used where there is a deficiency of anterosuperior rotator cuff, particularly in patients with recurrent anterior instability resulting from subscapularis insufficiency [74]. In the original description of the technique of pectoralis major tendon transfer from 1997 by Wirth et al., the upper portion of the pectoralis major tendon was transferred [75]. Resch described a technique in which the upper portion of the pectoralis major is rerouted underneath the conjoint tendon. In his opinion, this would give a more favourable line of action for the transfer compared with the traditional pectoralis major transfer [76]. To improve the line of action of the transferred pectoralis major without jeopardizing the musculoskeletal nerve, Warner modified the original pectoralis tendon transfer by rerouting its sternal head underneath the clavicular head before fixation to the lesser tuberosity (split pectoralis major transfer, SPM transfer) [77].

A slight modification of Warner technique was proposed by Gerber et al. Their tendon transfer combines the split pectoralis major tendon and the teres major tendon (SPM–TM transfer). The rationale of this combined tendon transfer is to replace the upper and lower portion of the subscapularis muscle with the split pectoralis major and teres major, respectively [78].

Recent literature confirms that pectorals major transfer is a safe and quite reliable procedure. In their systematic review of pectoralis major transfer in irreparable cuff tears, Shin et al. included eight studies with a total 195 shoulders. The mean follow-up was 33.4 months (range 6–80 months). Constant scores improved from a mean pre-operative score of 37.8 ± 6.8, to a mean postoperative score of 61.3 ± 6.5 ($p < 0.0001$). Although improvement in pain scores was impossible to assess due to different scores used, a trend in pain reduction was noted in all articles [79]. The Constant scores were significantly higher in patients following subcoracoid transfer of the pectoralis major tendon compared to patients who received supracoracoid transfer ($p < 0.001$). The overall reported incidence of postoperative nerve palsy is low (one transient musculocutaneous nerve palsy and one axillary nerve dysfunction out of 195 cases) [79].

It seems that pectoralis major transfers are a reasonable surgical option for the management of irreparable anterosuperior rotator cuff tears, particularly when the patient is experiencing anterior instability as a result of subscapularis insufficiency [41].

Latissimus dorsi transfer for a deficient superolateral and posterosuperior rotator cuff can produce a dramatic restoration of elevation of the shoulder. Transfer of the latissimus dorsi with or without the teres major has been known as a salvage procedure for irreparable superolateral rotator cuff tears since 1992, when it was first published by Gerber et al. [80]. It has been proved by many authors to be a valuable treatment option for painful or pain-free pseudoparalysis of external rotation provided that the subscapularis is intact. Results are better if there is no chronic pseudo paralysis of anterior elevation and if the teres minor does not show advanced fatty infiltration [1]. The ideal candidate is a patient who has maintained active anterior elevation, but lacks control of the arm in space in external rotation (simple weakness in external rotation is not a sufficient indication for surgery), and who also has an intact subscapularis and no glenohumeral arthritis [9]. Several surgical techniques have been used for latissimus dorsi transfer, including single-incision, double-incision, and more recently arthroscopically assisted transfer [41]. When it is transferred, the muscle no longer serves as an internal rotator but rather is an external rotator and humeral head depressor. A more posterior placement of the transfer on the greater tuberosity results in more external rotation, whereas more superior placement results in more humeral head depression [41]. Iannotti et al. [81] in there technique put patient in lateral decubitus position. A superior approach to the rotator cuff is achieved with detachment of the deltoid origin from the anterior aspect of the acromion and with a 4 cm split of the middle deltoid fibres. The coracoacromial ligament is taken off with the deltoid and is reattached at the conclusion of the operation. The bursa is excised, and the rotator cuff is inspected. All attempts are made to mobilize and repair the cuff. Acromioplasty is performed if needed. The subscapularis tear should be repaired if presents. A second incision is made along the lateral border of the latissimus dorsi to the posterior axillary crease. The latissimus dorsi insertion is identified with the arm abducted and internally rotated, and it is detached sharply from the humerus. The neurovascular pedicle is identified and protected, and the muscle is freed from its deep fascia attachments. A 1-mm Dacron suture is passed with use of a Krakow suture technique along each side of the tendon from the musculotendinous junction to the end of the tendon. Blunt dissection is performed to create a wide tunnel deep to the deltoid and superficial to the posterior cuff musculature. The latissimus dorsi muscle and tendon are brought over the top of the humeral head and are repaired anteriorly to the subscapularis, laterally to the greater tuberosity, and, if possible, medially to the torn retracted edges of the rotator cuff [81]. More recently arthroscopically assisted transfers have been reported. Arthroscopic assisted procedures can have a couple of advantages over open counterparts, one being easier identification and treatment of concomitant intraarticular pathologies [82].

In a systematic review of the literature performed by Namdari et al. results from 10 studies (258 patients, 262 shoulders) were compared. Patients were followed for a frequency-weighted mean of 45.5 months (range, 24–126 months). Frequency-weighted mean adjusted Constant score improved from 45.9 preoperatively to 73.2 postoperatively ($p < 0.001$). The frequency-weighted mean active forward elevation improved from 101.9° preoperatively to 137.4° postoperatively ($p < 0.001$), and the frequency-weighted mean active external rotation improved from 16.8° to 26.7° ($p < 0.001$). Authors found that subscapularis muscle insufficiency, advanced teres minor muscle atrophy, and the need for revision surgery were correlated with poor functional outcomes. The overall reported complication rate was 9.5% (25 of 262), which included among other seven cases of neuropraxia (2.7%) and nine tears of the transferred tendon(3.4%) [87].

In their long-term follow-up of minimum 10 years of 46 shoulders in 44 patients, Gerber et al. observed the mean subjective shoulder value (SSV) increase from 29% preoperatively to 70% at the time of final follow-up. The relative Constant score improved from 56 to 80, and the pain score improved from 7 to 13 points ($p < 0.0001$ for all). Mean flexion increased from 118° to 132°, abduction increased from 112° to 123°, and external rotation increased from 18° to 33°. Mean abduction strength increased from 1.2 to 2.0 kg ($p = 0.001$). There was a slight but significant increase in osteoarthritic changes. Inferior results occurred in shoulders with insufficiency of the subscapularis muscle and fatty infiltration of the teres minor muscle [84].

Latissmus dorsi transfer (with or without terms major) demonstrated to be a valuable option for improvement in shoulder function, range of motion, strength, and pain relief in patients with irreparable posterosuperior rotator cuff tears, however patients and physicians should not expect an outcome of 'normal' function or complete pain relief [83].

There is increased interest in using lower trapezius transfers for treatment of massive irreparable posterosuperior rotator cuff tears. Its use was first described by Elhassan et al. to improve external rotation in patients with brachial plexopathy [85]. A biomechanical investigation found that a lower trapezius transfer is more effective in restoring external rotation than the latissimus dorsi transfer [86]. In 2016 Elhassan et al. published their results of lower trapezius transfer with Achilles tendon augmentation at an average follow-up of 47 months [87]. All 32 patients had significant improvement in pain, subjective shoulder value, and shoulder range of motion [87]. Another relatively recent concept is the use of latissimus dorsi and teres major transfer in subscapularis insufficiency. The anatomic feasibility study of the latissimus dorsi (LD) with teres major (TM) muscle-tendon transfer to reconstruct an irreparable SS tendon tear by Elhassan et al. showed encouraging results [88].

5.2.4. Subacromial spacer

One of the most recent treatment modalities proposed for an irreparable rotator cuff tears is the use of a subacromial balloon or spacer [89]. The most commonly used balloon system which contains an introducer and a presbaped spacer (available in 3 different sizes) made of poly(L-lactide-co-caprolactone), which is a copolymer of poly-lactide and -caprolactone. This is a biodegradable and widely used material that dissolves over a period of 12 months [45]. It is unclear, however, how long the spacer remains inflated. The spacer works by reducing subacromial friction through lowering the humeral head during abduction [89]. To enable insertion, the balloon is folded into a cylinder-shaped insertion tube, which is removed once the spacer is inserted into the subacromial space [89]. After a standard arthroscopy including debridement and bursectomy, the rotator cuff is assessed for reparability. Once deemed irreparable, the correct size of the spacer must be chosen. The biodegradable spacer is introduced through the lateral port and is inflated with saline to its maximal volume depending on the spacer size. As a final step, the delivery system is removed, and the shoulder is passively moved through a full range of movement to verify that the spacer is accurately placed, is stable in position, and does not interfere with shoulder mobility [89]. This balloon can be used in patients with irreparable tears of SST and IST. It is recommended to repair the subscapularis to create anterior-posterior coupling. Contraindications include glenohumeral arthropathy, active infection and allergy to device material.

Senekovic et al. published their 5 year follow-up of 24 patients who were treated with a balloon device. Of the participating subjects who reached the 5-year follow-up, 84.6% of the patients showed a clinically significant improvement of at least 15 points in Constant score, while 61.54% showed at least 25 points of improvement. Only 10% of the treated patients showed no improvement or worsening in the shoulder score comparing to their baseline. Further randomized controlled trials in larger cohorts are needed [90].

5.2.5. Superior capsule reconstruction

The shoulder capsule is an important static stabilizer of the glenohumeral joint [91]. The anterior capsule serves to maintain glenohumeral stability anteriorly, whereas posterior capsule plays an important role with posterior stability [8, 91]. The superior capsule attaches to a significant portion of the greater tuberosity, with an anatomic study indicating a range between 30% and 61% of total surface area [92]. As a result, it is often disrupted when complete tears of the supraspinatus or infraspinatus occur [41]. A recent biomechanical study determined that superior capsular defects led to increased glenohumeral translation in all directions, particularly with superior translation at 5 and 30° of abduction [91]. Mihata et al. developed arthroscopic superior capsule reconstruction (ASCR) [93] to restore superior stability of the shoulder joint of patient with irreparable cuff tears [93, 94].

Arthroscopic subacromial decompression and debridement of both the superior glenoid and rotator cuff footprint of the greater tuberosity is performed. If torn, the subscapularis tendon should be repaired and a partial repair of a torn infraspinatus and teres minor tendons is advised. The size of the superior capsular defect is evaluated. Then a graft 6–8 mm thick is prepared and inserted into the subacromial space through the lateral portal. It is then attached to the superior glenoid by using 2 suture anchors inserted into the superior glenoid. The lateral side of the graft is attached to the rotator cuff footprint on the greater tuberosity by using a compression double-row technique [93]. Finally, side-to-side sutures between the graft and the infraspinatus tendon and between the graft and the residual anterior supraspinatus tendon or subscapularis tendon are added to improve force coupling in the shoulder joint. Careful attention should be paid to overtightening of the side-to-side suture on the anterior side to avoid shoulder contracture after surgery [93].

In their group of 23 patients (24 shoulder), Mihata et al. [93] reported improvement of mean active elevation from 84 to 148 ($p < 0.001$) and of external rotation from 26 to 40 ($p < 0.01$). Acromiohumeral distance (AHD) increased from 4.6 ± 2.2 mm preoperatively to 8.7 ± 2.6 mm postoperatively ($p < 0.0001$). There were no cases of progression of osteoarthritis or rotator cuff muscle atrophy. Twenty patients (83.3%) had no graft tear or tendon retear during follow-up (24–51 months). The American Shoulder and Elbow Surgeons (ASES) score improved from 23.5 to 92.9 points ($p < 0.0001$). These encouraging results suggest that this reconstruction technique useful alternative treatment for irreparable rotator cuff tears. Human dermal allograft has been also successfully used in this procedure [72].

5.2.6. Rotator cuff repair with patch

As previously mentioned, cuff repair in massive tears is a complicated task. Retear rates are high, and depending on the source may reach 34–94% [10]. What is interesting is that patients who undergo repair which subsequently fail, still show improved functional outcomes postoperatively [95–97]. However, their results are worse than in those where healing was achieved [98, 99]. In an attempt to decrease the failure rate and improve the outcomes of massive cuff tears repair, the use of patch grafts was introduced and popularized by various authors. Many varieties of patch materials have been developed and used clinically, including synthetic materials Polyester ligament (Dacron) [100], Gore-Tex soft tissue patch [101], Mersilene mesh [102], Teflon felt [103] and Carbon fibrebre patches [104], allografts freeze*dried rotator cuff [105, 106], quadriceps tendon [107], patellar tendon, achilles tendon [107], dermal matrix (Graftjacket) [107], tensor fascia late [108] and xenografts porcine dermal collagen [109, 110], porcine small intestinal submucosa [111]. Autografts such as the biceps tendon [112, 113] and tensor fascia late [114] have also been used. Patch reinforcement can be performed as augmentation (onlay) of a cuff repair, in which the rotator cuff is repaired to nearly normal status and patch is then either implemented into the repair construct or sutured over the top of the repaired tendon [99]. The other method is interposition (intercalary), wherein the graft bridges the gap between the irreparable cuff edge and cuff footprint on the humerus [99]. As the use of patches for massive cuff tears repair is a subject of a great deal of interest, much has been published throughout last 20 years. Unfortunately most of the reports are case reports or short term case series on a relatively small groups of patients. Each of these studies typically represents the experience of one surgeon or one institution and therefore, when taken alone, may not be an accurate reflection of patch use more broadly. Comprehensive reviews can provide valuable summarized data, giving clinicians a broader picture on this interesting topic. A recent review was performed by Steinhaus et al. in 2016 [99]. They reviewed results of 24 studies, published between 1986 and 2014. The frequency-weighted mean age of patients was 61.9 years with 35.4 months' follow-up. There were a total of 566 patients included. The most common surgical technique used across the 24 studies was open patch repair, representing 54.6% of cases (309 of 566), followed by mini-open in 170 cases and arthroscopic in 87 cases. The most common graft source was synthetic, representing 44.3% of grafts (251 of 566), followed by allograft in 188 cases and xenograft in 127 cases. The graft was used to bridge the gap between the retracted cuff and humerus (interposition) in 56.3% of patients (319 of 566), whereas it was used to augment the repair in 43.6% (247 of 566). Augmentation and interposition techniques showed similar improvements in range of motion, strength, and patient-reported outcomes (PROs), pain and activities of daily living (ADLs) whereas xenografts showed less improvement in PROs and ADLs compared with other graft types. The overall retear rate was 25%, with rates of 34% and 12% for augmentation and interposition, respectively, and rates of 44%, 23%, and 15% for xenografts, allografts, and synthetic grafts, respectively.

In summary, all studies showed improvements in clinical and functional outcomes, without much difference between augmentation and interposition techniques. Xenografts seem to do worse than allografts and synthetic materials. What is interesting and might be counterintuitive for many, is the fact that retear rate was lower with the interposition technique. Of course systemic reviews are only as good as the studies they are based on, so as promising as the results seem to be, there is no doubt that patch grafting needs well designed prospective comparison studies to truly assess its value in massive cuff tears treatment.

6. Leeds Cuff Patch

Our technique of choice in surgical treatment of irreparable rotator cuff tear was developed by the senior author. We utilize a non-absorbable polyester patch which is sutured over the torn rotator cuff. It thus provides reinforcement of incompletely repaired rotator cuff tears and those at high risk of re-tear due to poor quality soft tissue. It can be used both as a bridging graft and augmentation. Leeds Cuff Patch a synthetic patch that is indicated for reconstruction of chronic massive, full thickness rotator cuff tears where the retracted tear cannot be mobilized back to the bony attachment site or where the cuff tissue has undergone degeneration. The patch implant is produced from polyethylene terephthalate (PET), commonly known as polyester. This is a non-absorbable biocompatible material that has been in use for the reconstruction of ligaments and tendons for over 25 years. The design of the patch comprises a base component with an integral reinforcement component. The base component has a 'open structure' that acts as a scaffold allowing tissue ingrowth. The reinforcement provides enhanced strength to the patch. The patch can be implanted with typical techniques and sutures as used for other tendon augmentation xenograft and allograft patches. The weak point of a repair with such products is between the suture and tendon. However, the integral reinforcement of the patch provides resistance to suture pull-through and thus addresses this common failure mode for such devices.

Conducting our own research, we compared outcomes of the Leeds Cuff Patch with other treatment interventions available (e.g. anterior deltoid rehabilitation exercises, arthroscopic rotator cuff repair, arthroscopic rotator cuff debridement) for patients with large or massive cuff tears.

We recruited 68 patients with large and massive rotator cuff tears: 29 in the Patch group and 39 as controls. The treatment decision was made based on patient choice and intra-operative findings: those patients who wished to avoid operative intervention underwent anterior deltoid rehabilitation; those with arthroscopically reparable tears received that treatment; those with arthroscopically irreparable tears but mobile cuff underwent open patch repair; those with substantial retraction of poor quality immobile tendon underwent debridement. All patients completed Oxford Shoulder Score (OSS), Shoulder Pain and Disability Index (SPADI), and Constant score at baseline, 6 weeks and 6 months following treatment.

The Patch group demonstrated improvement in all outcomes from baseline to 6 months (paired mean difference OSS 12.3, SPADI 18.8, Constant 13.9), as did the Control group (paired mean difference OSS 8.7, SPADI 18.8, Constant 11.1). When the patients with very poor quality rotator cuff were removed, the results were OSS 14.3 SPADI Constant 18.0. The arthroscopically repaired group showed very similar results to the remainder of the controls. Those with better quality tendon but still non-repairable had a clinically significant improvement in OSS compared with the non-patch group.

We are extending the follow-up period for this study to 2 years, and will also analyse MRI scans performed at baseline, 6 months and 2 years following surgery. This will provide both clinical and radiological outcomes of patch repair of large and massive rotator cuff tears, and be one of the first studies comparing patches with other treatment options for this group of patients.

7. Summary

There are a wide variety of options available to surgeon for the patient with a large to massive tear of the rotator cuff causing pain and loss of function. Most of these have been reported as having quite reasonable outcomes in the published literature. In the UK, less than 30% of upper limb surgeons, would consider a patch, and further research is required. Newer procedures such as superior capsular reconstruction and balloon arthroplasty warrant further investigation. Reverse TSR gives excellent outcomes in the older patient, but for younger patients with large or massive rotator cuff tears, though there are a number of surgical options available, the evidence to support each needs strengthening with further research into this exciting area of shoulder surgery.

Author details

Roger Hackney[1]*, Piotr Lesniewski[2] and Paul Cowling[2]

*Address all correspondence to: rogerhackney@hotmail.com

1 Spire Hospital, Leeds, United Kingdom

2 Chapel Allerton Hospital LTH, Leeds, United Kingdom

References

[1] Gerber C, Wirth SH, Farshad M. Treatment options for massive rotator cuff tears. Journal of Shoulder and Elbow Surgery. 2011;**20**:S20-S29

[2] Guery J, Favard L, Sirveaux F, Oudet D, Mole D, Walch G. Reverse total shoulder arthroplasty. Survivorship analysis of eighty replacements followed for five to ten years. Journal of Bone and Joint Surgery. American Volume. 2006;**88**:1742-1747

[3] 13th Annual Report 2016 National Joint Registry for England, Wales, Northern Ireland and the Isle of Man Surgical data to 31 December 2015. p. 26,170, njrcentre.org.uk

[4] Burkhart SS, Danaceau SM, Pearce CE Jr. Arthroscopic rotator cuff repair: Analysis of results by tear size and by repair technique-margin convergence versus direct tendon-to-bone repair. Arthroscopy. 2001;**17**:905-912

[5] Lo IK, Burkhart SS. Arthroscopic revision of failed rotator cuff repairs: Technique and results. Arthroscopy. 2004;**20**:250-267

[6] Cofield RH. Subscapular muscle transposition for repair of chronic rotator cuff tears. Surgery, Gynecology & Obstetrics. 1982;**154**:667-672

[7] Davidson J, Burkhart SS. The geometric classification of rotator cuff tears: A system linking tear pattern to treatment and prognosis. Arthroscopy. 2010;**26**:417-424

[8] Gerber C, Fuchs B, Hodler J. The results of repair of massive tears of the rotator cuff. The Journal of Bone and Joint Surgery. American Volume. 2000;**82**:505-515

[9] Lädermann A, Denard PJ, Collin P. Massive rotator cuff tears: Definition and treatment. International Orthopaedics (SICOT). 2015;**39**:2403-2414

[10] Neri BR, Chan KW, Kwon YW. Management of massive and irreparable rotator cuff tears. Journal of Shoulder and Elbow Surgery. 2009;**18**:808-818

[11] Jeong JY et al. Comparison of outcomes with arthroscopic repair of acute-on-chronic within 6 months and chronic rotator cuff tears. Journal of Shoulder and Elbow Surgery. 2017;**26**(4):648-655

[12] Warner JJ, Gerber C. Treatment of massive rotator cuff tears: Posterior-superior and anterior-superior. Rosemont, IL: American Academy of Orthopaedic Surgeons; 1998

[13] Collin P, Matsumura N, Lädermann A, Denard PJ, Walch G. Relationship between massive chronic rotator cuff tear pattern and loss of active shoulder range of motion. Journal of Shoulder and Elbow Surgery. 2014;**23**(8):1195-1202

[14] Goutallier D, Postel JM, Lavau L, Bernageau J. Influence de la d eg en erescence graisseuse des muscles supra epineux et infra epineux sur le pronostic des r eparations chirurgicales de la coiffe des rotateurs. Rev Chir Orthop. 1999;**85**:668-676

[15] Walch G, Boulahia A, Calderone S, Robinson AH. The 'dropping' and 'hornblower's' signs in evaluation of rotator-cuff tears. Journal of Bone and Joint Surgery. British Volume (London). 1998;**80**:624-628

[16] Goutallier D, Postel JM, Bernageau J, Lavau L, Voisin MC. Fatty muscle degeneration in cuff ruptures. Pre- and postoperative evaluation by CT scan. Clinical Orthopaedics and Related Research. 1994;**304**:78-83

[17] Gladstone JN, Bishop JY, Lo IK, Flatow EL. Fatty infiltration and atrophy of the rotator cuff do not improve after rotator cuff repair and correlate with poor functional outcome. The American Journal of Sports Medicine. 2007;**35**:719-728

[18] Sher JS, Uribe JW, Posada A, Murphy BJ, Zlatkin MB. Abnormal findings on magnetic resonance images of asymptomatic shoulders. The Journal of Bone and Joint Surgery. American Volume. 1995;**77**:10-15

[19] Gerber C, Galantay RV, Hersche O. The pattern of pain produced by irritation of the acromioclavicular joint and the subacromial space. Journal of Shoulder and Elbow Surgery. 1998;**7**:352-355

[20] Gerber C, Blumenthal S, Curt A, Werner CM. Effect of selective experimental suprascapular nerve block on abduction and external rotation strength of the shoulder. J Shoulder Elbow Surg. 2007;**16**:815-820

[21] Werner CM, Steinmann PA, Gilbart M, Gerber C. Treatment of painful pseudoparalysis due to irreparable rotator cuff dysfunction with the Delta III reverse-ball-and-socket total shoulder prosthesis. The Journal of Bone and Joint Surgery. American Volume. 2005;**87**:1476-1486

[22] Denard PJ, Lädermann A, Jiwani AZ, Burkhart SS. Functional outcome after arthroscopic repair of massive rotator cuff tears in individuals with pseudoparalysis. Arthroscopy. 2012;**28**:1214-1219

[23] Tokish JM, Decker MJ, Ellis HB, Torry MR, Hawkins RJ. The belly-press test for the physical examination of the subscapularis muscle: Electromyographic validation and comparison to the lift-off test. Journal of Shoulder and Elbow Surgery. 2003;**12**:427-430

[24] Weiner DS, Macnab I. Superior migration of the humeral head. A radiological aid in the diagnosis of tears of the rotator cuff. Journal of Bone and Joint Surgery. British Volume (London). 1970;**52**:524-527

[25] Walch G, Marechal E, Maupas J, Liotard JP. Surgical treatment of rotator cuff rupture. Prognostic factors [in French]. Revue de Chirurgie Orthopédique et Réparatrice de l'Appareil Moteur. 1992;**78**:379-388

[26] Hamada K, Yamanaka K, Yetal U. A radiographic classification of massive rotator cuff tear arthritis. Clinical Orthopaedics and Related Research. 2011;**469**:2452-2460

[27] Iannotti JP, Zlatkin MB, Esterhai JL, Kressel HY, Dalinka MK, Spindler KP. Magnetic resonance imaging of the shoulder. Sensitivity, specificity, and predictive value. The Journal of Bone and Joint Surgery. American Volume. 1991;**73**:17-29

[28] Fuchs B, Weishaupt D, Zanetti M, Hodler J, Gerber C. Fatty degeneration of the muscles of the rotator cuff: Assessment by computed tomography versus magnetic resonance imaging. Journal of Shoulder and Elbow Surgery. 1999;**8**:599-605

[29] Zanetti M, Gerber C, Hodler J. Quantitative assessment of the muscles of the rotator cuff with magnetic resonance imaging. Investigative Radiology. 1998;**33**:163-170

[30] Williams MD, Lädermann A, Melis B, Barthelemy R, Walch G. Fatty infiltration of the supraspinatus: A reliability study. Journal of Shoulder and Elbow Surgery. 2009;**18**:581-587

[31] Kissenberth MJ, Rulewicz GJ, Hamilton SC, Bruch HE, Hawkins RJ. A positive tangent sign predicts the repairability of rotator cuff tears. Journal of Shoulder and Elbow Surgery. 2014;**23**:1023-1027

[32] Kim JY, Park JS, Rhee YG. Can preoperative magnetic resonance imaging predict the reparability of massive rotator cuff tears? Am J Sports Med. 2017;**45**:1654-1663

[33] Teefey SA, Rubin DA, Middleton WD, Hildebolt CF, Leibold RA, Yamaguchi K. Detection and quantification of rotator cuff tears. Comparison of ultrasonographic, magnetic resonance imaging, and arthroscopic findings in seventy-one consecutive cases. Journal of Bone and Joint Surgery. American Volume. 2004;**86**:708-716

[34] Zingg PO, Jost B, Sukthankar A, Buhler M, Pfirrmann CW, Gerber C. Clinical and structural outcomes of nonoperative management of massive rotator cuff tears. The Journal of Bone and Joint Surgery. American Volume. 2007;**89**:1928-1934

[35] Williams GR Jr, Rockwood CA Jr. Hemiarthroplasty in rotator cuff-deficient shoulders. Journal of Shoulder and Elbow Surgery. 1996;**5**:362-367

[36] Koester MC et al. The efficacy of subacromial corticosteroid injection in the treatment of rotator cuff disease: A systematic review. The Journal of the American Academy of Orthopaedic Surgeons. 2007;**15**(1):3-11

[37] Shibata Y, Midorikawa K, Emoto G, Naito M. Clinical evaluation of sodium hyaluronate for the treatment of patients with rotator cuff tear. Journal of Shoulder and Elbow Surgery. 2001;**10**:209-216

[38] Funk L, Haines J, Trail I. Rotator cuff arthropathy. Current Orthopaedics. 2007;**21**:415-421

[39] Funk L. Ostenil hyaluronan for inoperable osteoarthritis of the shoulder. Osteoarthritis Cartilage. 2004;**12**(Suppl. B):140

[40] Grammont PM, Baulot E. Delta shoulder prosthesis for rotator cuff rupture. Orthopedics. 1993;**16**:65-68

[41] Greenspoon JA, Petri M, Warth RJ, Millett PJ. Massive rotator cuff tears: Pathomechanics, current treatment options, and clinical outcomes. Journal of Shoulder and Elbow Surgery. 2015;**24**:1493-1505

[42] Kane TP, Rogers P, Hazelgrove J, Wimsey S, Harper GD. Pulsed radiofrequency applied to the suprascapular nerve in painful cuff tear arthropathy. Journal of Shoulder and Elbow Surgery. 2008;**17**:436-440

[43] Aszmann OC, Dellon AL, Birely BT, McFarland EG. Innervation of the human shoulder joint and its implications for surgery. Clinical Orthopaedics and Related Research. 1996;**330**:202-207

[44] Emery P, Bowman S, Wedderburn L, Grahame R. Suprascapular nerve block for chronic shoulder pain in rheumatoid arthritis. BMJ. 1989;**299**:1079-1080

[45] Anley CM, Chan SKL, Snow M. Arthroscopic treatment options for irreparable rotator cuff tears of the shoulder. World Journal of Orthopedics. 2014;**5**(5):557-565

[46] Nizlan NM, Skirving AP, Campbell PT. Arthroscopic suprascapular neurectomy for the management of severe shoulder pain. Journal of Shoulder and Elbow Surgery. 2009;**18**:245-250

[47] Klinger HM, Spahn G, Baums MH, Steckel H. Arthroscopic debridement of irreparable massive rotator cuff tearsda comparison of debridement alone and combined procedure with biceps tenotomy. Acta Chirurgica Belgica. 2005;**105**:297-230

[48] Liem D, Alci S, Dedy N, Steinbeck J, Marquardt B, Möllenhoff G. Clinical and structural results of partial supraspinatus tears treated by subacromial decompression without repair. Knee Surgery, Sports Traumatology, Arthroscopy. 2008;**16**:967-972

[49] Melillo AS, Savoie FH III, Field LD. Massive rotator cuff tears: Debridement versus repair. The Orthopedic Clinics of North America. 1997;**28**:117-124

[50] Burkhart S, Lo I, Brady P. A cowboy's guide to advanced shoulder arthroscopy. Philadelphia: Lippincott Williams & Wilkins; 2006. p. 81 84-87, 89-91

[51] Lädermann A, Chague S, Kolo FC, Charbonnier C. Kinematics of the shoulder joint in tennis players. Journal of Science and Medicine in Sport. 2016;**19**:56-63

[52] Kim JR, Ryu KJ, Hong IT, Kim BK, Kim JH. Can a high acromion index predict rotator cuff tears? International Orthopaedics. 2012;**36**:1019-1024

[53] Moor BK, Wieser K, Slankamenac K, Gerber C, Bouaicha S. Relationship of individual scapular anatomy and degenerative rotator cuff tears. Journal of Shoulder and Elbow Surgery. 2014;**23**:536-541

[54] Rockwood CA Jr, Williams GR Jr, Burkhead WZ Jr. Debridement of degenerative, irreparable lesions of the rotator cuff. The Journal of Bone and Joint Surgery. American Volume. 1995;**77**:857-866

[55] Gartsman GM. Massive, irreparable tears of the rotator cuff. Results of operative debridement and subacromial decompression. The Journal of Bone and Joint Surgery. American Volume. 1997;**79**:715-721

[56] Scheibel M, Lichtenberg S, Habermeyer P. Reversed arthroscopic subacromial decompression for massive rotator cuff tears. Journal of Shoulder and Elbow Surgery. 2004; **13**:272-278

[57] Fenlin JM, Chase JM, Rushton SA, Frieman BG. Tuberoplasty: Creation of an acromiohumeral articulation-a treatment option for massive, irreparable rotator cuff tears. Journal of Shoulder and Elbow Surgery. 2002;**11**:136-142

[58] Verhelst L, Vandekerckhove PJ, Sergeant G, Liekens K, Van Hoonacker P, Berghs B. Reversed arthroscopic subacromial decompression for symptomatic irreparable rotator cuff tears: Mid-term follow-up results in 34 shoulders. Journal of Shoulder and Elbow Surgery. 2010;**19**:601-608

[59] Lee BG, Cho NS, Rhee YG. Results of arthroscopic decompression and tuberoplasty for irreparable massive rotator cuff tears. Arthroscopy. 2011;**27**:1341-1350

[60] Walch G, Madonia G, Pozzi I, Riand N, Levigne C. Arthroscopic tenotomy of the long head of the biceps in rotator cuff ruptures. In: Gazielly DF, Gleyze P, Thomas T, editors. The cuff. Paris: Elsevier; 1997. p. 350-355

[61] Pagnani MJ, Deng XH, Warren RF, Torzilli PA, O'Brien SJ. Role of the long head of the biceps brachii in glenohumeral stability: A biomechanical study in cadavera. Journal of Shoulder and Elbow Surgery. 1996;**5**:255-262

[62] Walch G, Edwards TB, Boulahia A, Nove-Josserand L, Neyton L, Szabo I. Arthroscopic tenotomy of the long head of the biceps in the treatment of rotator cuff tears: Clinical and radiographic results of 307 cases. Journal of Shoulder and Elbow Surgery. 2005;**14**:238e6

[63] Kempf JF, Gleyze P, Bonnomet F, Walch G, Mole D, Frank A, et al. A multicenter study of 210 rotator cuff tears treated by arthroscopic acromioplasty. Arthroscopy. 1999;**15**:56-66

[64] Walch G, Edwards TB, Boulahia A, Nove-Josserand L, Neyton L, Szabo I. Arthroscopic tenotomy of the long head of the biceps in the treatment of rotator cuff tears: Clinical and radiographic results of 307 cases. Journal of Shoulder and Elbow Surgery. 2005;**14**:238-246

[65] Wuelker N, Plitz W, Roetman B. Biomechanical data concerning the shoulder impingement syndrome. Clinical Orthopaedics and Related Research. 1994:242-249

[66] Flatow EL, Soslowsky LJ, Ticker JB, Pawluk RJ, Hepler M, Ark J, et al. Excursion of the rotator cuff under the acromion. Patterns of subacromial contact. The American Journal of Sports Medicine. 1994;**22**:779-788

[67] LS O, Wolf BR, Hall MP, Levy BA, Marx RG. Indications for rotator cuff repair: A systematic review. Clinical Orthopaedics and Related Research. 2007;**455**:52-63

[68] Cofield RH, Parvizi J, Hoffmeyer PJ, Lanzer WL, Ilstrup DM, Rowland CM. Surgical repair of chronic rotator cuff tears. A prospective long-term study. Journal of Bone and Joint Surgery. American Volume. 2001;**83**:71

[69] Burkhart SS, Nottage WM, Ogilvie-Harris DJ, Kohn HS, Pachelli A. Partial repair of irreparable rotator cuff tears. Arthroscopy. 1994;**10**:363-370

[70] Gerber C, Schneeberger AG, Beck M, Schlegel U. Mechanical strength of repairs of the rotator cuff. Journal of Bone and Joint Surgery. British Volume (London). 1994;**76**:371-380

[71] Gerber C, Schneeberger AG, Perren SM, Nyffeler RW. Experimental rotator cuff repair. A preliminary study. The Journal of Bone and Joint Surgery. American Volume. 1999;**81**:1281-1290

[72] Thorsness R, Romeo A. Massive rotator cuff tears: Trends in surgical management. Trending in Orthopedics. 2016;**39**:145-51

[73] Warner JJ. Management of massive irreparable rotator cuff tears: The role of tendon transfer. Instructional Course Lectures. 2001;**50**:63-71

[74] Galatz LM, Connor PM, Calfee RP, Hsu JC, Yamaguchi K. Pectoralis major transfer for anterior-superior subluxation in massive rotator cuff insufficiency. Journal of Shoulder and Elbow Surgery. 2003;**12**:1-5

[75] Wirth MA, Rockwood CA Jr. Operative treatment of irreparable rupture of the subscapularis. The Journal of Bone and Joint Surgery. American Volume. 1997;**79-5**:722-731

[76] Resch H, Povacz P, Ritter E, et al. Transfer of the pectoralis major muscle for the treatment of irreparable rupture of the subscapularis tendon. The Journal of Bone and Joint Surgery. American Volume. 2000;**82**(3):372-382

[77] Warner J. Management of massive irreparable rotator cuff tears: The role of tendon transfers. Instructional course lec tures. Journal of Bone and Joint Surgery. American Volume. 2001;**50**:63-71

[78] Gerber A, Clavert P, Millett PJ, Holovacs TF, Warner JJP. Split pectoralis major and teres major tendon transfers for massive irreparable tears of the susbcapularis. Techniques in Shoulder and Elbow Surgery. 2004;**5**:5-12

[79] Shin JJ, Saccomanno MF, Cole BJ, Romeo AA, Nicholson GP, Verma NN. Pectoralis major transfer for treatment of irreparable subscapularis tear: A systematic review. Knee Surgery, Sports Traumatology, Arthroscopy. 2016;**24**:1951-60

[80] Gerber C, Vinh TS, Hertel R, Hess CW. Latissimus dorsi transfer for the treatment of massive tears of the rotator cuff. A preliminary report. Clinical Orthopaedics and Related Research. 1988:51-61

[81] Iannotti JP, Hennigan S, Herzog R, Kella S, Kelley M, Leggin B, Williams GR. Latissimus dorsi tendon transfer for irreparable posterosuperior rotator cuff tears. The Journal of Bone & Joint Surgery. 2006;**88**(2);342-348

[82] Jermolajevas V, Kordasiewicz B. Arthroscopically assisted latissimus dorsi tendon transfer in beach-chair position. Arthroscopy Techniques. 2015;**4**(4):e359-e363

[83] Namdari S, Voleti P, Baldwin K, Glasser D, Huffman GR. Latissimus dorsi tendon transfer for irreparable rotator cuff tears: A systematic review. The Journal of Bone and Joint Surgery. American Volume. 2012;**94**:891-898

[84] Gerber C, Rahm SA, Catanzaro S, Farshad M, Moor BK. Latissimus dorsi tendon transfer for treatment of irreparable posterosuperior rotator cuff tears: Long-term results at a minimum follow-up of ten years. The Journal of Bone and Joint Surgery. American Volume. 2013;**95**:1920-1926

[85] Elhassan B, Bishop A, Shin A. Trapezius transfer to restore external rotation in a patient with a brachial plexus injury. A case report. The Journal of Bone and Joint Surgery. American Volume. 2009;**91**:263-267

[86] Hartzler RU, Barlow JD, An KN, Elhassan BT. Biomechanical effectiveness of different types of tendon transfers to the shoulder for external rotation. Journal of Shoulder and Elbow Surgery. 2012;**21**:1370-1376

[87] Elhassan BT, Wagner ER, Werthel J-D. Outcome of lower trapezius transfer to reconstruct massive irreparable posterior-superior rotator cuff tear. Journal of Shoulder and Elbow Surgery. 2016;**25**:1346-1353

[88] Elhassan B, Christensen TJ, Wagner ER. Feasibility of latissimus and teres major transfer to reconstruct irreparable subscapularis tendon tear: An anatomic study. Journal of Shoulder and Elbow Surgery. 2014;**23**:492-499

[89] Savarese E, Romeo R. New solution for massive, irreparable rotator cuff tears: The subacromial "biodegradable spacer". Arthroscopy Techniques. 2012;**1**:e69-e74

[90] Senekovic V, Poberaj B, Kovacic L, Mikek M, Adar E, Markovitz E, Maman E, Dekel A. The biodegradable spacer as a novel treatment modality for massive rotator cuff tears: A prospective study with 5-year follow-up. Archives of Orthopaedic and Trauma Surgery. 2017;**137**:95-103

[91] Ishihara Y, Mihata T, Tamboli M, Nguyen L, Park KJ, McGarry MH, et al. Role of the superior shoulder capsule in passive stability of the glenohumeral joint. Journal of Shoulder and Elbow Surgery. 2014;**23**:642-648

[92] Nimura A, Kato A, Yamaguchi K, Mochizuki T, Okawa A, Sugaya H, et al. The superior capsule of the shoulder joint complements the insertion of the rotator cuff. Journal of Shoulder and Elbow Surgery. 2012;**21**:867-872

[93]   Mihata T, Lee TQ, Watanabe C, Fukunishi K, Ohue M, Tsujimura T, et al. Clinical results of arthroscopic superior capsule reconstruction for irreparable rotator cuff tears. Arthroscopy. 2013;**29**:459-470

[94]   Mihata T, McGarry MH, Pirolo JM, Kinoshita M, Lee TQ. Superior capsular reconstruction to restore superior stability in irreparable rotator cuff tears: A biomechanical and cadaveric study. The American Journal of Sports Medicine. 2012;**38**:369-374

[95]   Jost B, Pfirrmann CW, Gerber C, Switzerland Z. Clinical outcome after structural failure of rotator cuff repairs. The Journal of Bone and Joint Surgery. American Volume. 2000;**82**:304-314

[96]   Klepps S, Bishop J, Lin J, et al. Prospective evaluation of the effect of rotator cuff integrity on the outcome of open rotator cuff repairs. The American Journal of Sports Medicine. 2004;**32**:1716-1722

[97]   Liu SH, Baker CL. Arthroscopically assisted rotator cuff repair: Correlation of functional results with integrity of the cuff. Arthroscopy. 1994;**10**:54-60

[98]   Slabaugh MA, Nho SJ, Grumet RC, et al. Does the literature confirm superior clinical results in radiographically healed rotator cuffs after rotator cuff repair? Arthroscopy. 2010;**26**:393-403

[99]   Steinhaus ME, Makhni EC, Cole BJ, Romeo AA, Verma NN. Outcomes after patch use in rotator cuff repair. Arthroscopy. 2016;**32**:1676-90

[100] Nada AN, Debnath UK, Robinson DA, Jordan C. Treatment of massive rotator-cuff tears with a polyester ligament (Dacron) augmentation: Clinical outcome. Journal of Bone and Joint Surgery. British Volume (London). 2010;**92**:1397-1402 PMID: 20884978

[101] Hirooka A, Yoneda M, Wakaitani S, Isaka Y, Hayashida K, Fukushima S, Okamura K. Augmentation with a Gore-Tex patch for repair of large rotator cuff tears that cannot be sutured. Journal of Orthopaedic Science. 2002;**7**:451-456

[102] Audenaert E, Van Nuffel J, Schepens A, Verhelst M, Verdonk R. Reconstruction of massive rotator cuff lesions with a synthetic interposition graft: A prospective study of 41 patients. Knee Surgery, Sports Traumatology, Arthroscopy. 2006;**14**:360-364

[103] Ozaki J, Fujimoto S, Masuhara K, Tamai S, Yoshimoto S. Reconstruction of chronic massive rotator cuff tears with synthetic materials. Clinical Orthopaedics and Related Research. 1986;(202):173-183

[104] Visuri T, Kiviluoto O, Eskelin M. Carbon ber for repair of the rotator cuff. A 4-year follow-up of 14 cases. Acta Orthopaedica Scandinavica. 1991;**62**:356-359

[105] Nasca RJ. The use of freeze-dried allografts in the management of global rotator cuff tears. Clinical Orthopaedics and Related Research. 1988;(228):218-226

[106] Bond JL, Dopirak RM, Higgins J, Burns J, Snyder SJ. Arthroscopic replacement of massive, irreparable rotator cuff tears using a GraftJacket allograft: Technique and preliminary results. Arthroscopy. 2008;**24**:403-409 e1

[107] Moore DR, Cain EL, Schwartz ML, Clancy WG. Allograft reconstruction for massive, irreparable rotator cuff tears. The American Journal of Sports Medicine. 2006;**34**:392-396

[108] Ito J, Morioka T. Surgical treatment for large and massive tears of the rotator cuff. International Orthopaedics. 2003;**27**:228-231

[109] Badhe SP, Lawrence TM, Smith FD, Lunn PG. An assessment of porcine dermal xeno-graft as an augmentation graft in the treatment of extensive rotator cuff tears. Journal of Shoulder and Elbow Surgery. 2008;**17**:35S-39S

[110] Soler JA, Gidwani S, Curtis MJ. Early complications from the use of porcine dermal col-lagen implants (Permacol) as bridging constructs in the repair of massive rotator cuff tears. A report of 4 cases. Acta Orthopaedica Belgica. 2007;**73**:432-436

[111] Iannotti JP, Codsi MJ, Kwon YW, Derwin K, Ciccone J, Brems JJ. Porcine small intestine submucosa augmentation of surgical repair of chronic two-tendon rotator cuff tears. A randomized, controlled trial. Journal of Bone and Joint Surgery. American volume. 2006;**88**:1238-1244

[112] Sano H, Mineta M, Kita A, Itoi E. Tendon patch grafting using the long head of the biceps for irreparable massive rotator cuff tears. Journal of Orthopaedic Science. 2010; **15**:310-316

[113] Rhee YG, Cho NS, Lim CT, Yi JW, Vishvanathan T. Bridging the gap in immobile mas-sive rotator cuff tears: Augmentation using the tenotomized biceps. The American Journal of Sports Medicine. 2008;**36**:1511-1518

[114] Mori D, Funakoshi N, Yamashita F. Arthroscopic surgery of irreparable large or mas-sive rotator cuff tears with low-grade fatty degeneration of the infraspinatus: Patch autograft procedure versus partial repair procedure. Arthroscopy. 2013;**29**:1911-1921

5

Complete Rotator Cuff Tear: An Evidence-Based Conservative Management Approach

Taiceer A. Abdulwahab, William D. Murrell,
Frank Z. Jenio, Navneet Bhangra,
Gerard A. Malanga, Michael Stafford,
Nitin B. Jain and Olivier Verborgt

Abstract

Rotator cuff disease accounts for 10% of all shoulder pain and major shoulder disability, with limited information concerning the natural history and treatment approaches for the disorder. Our objective is to assess the available evidence for the efficacy and morbidity of commonly used systemic medications, physiotherapy, and injections alongside evaluating any negative long-term effects. Although there is conflicting literature, there appears to be some consensus on the best indicators for choosing to treat a full-thickness tears (FTT) non-operatively to reduce pain and improve function. The risks associated with these tears include the potential of the progression of the tear, a diminished healing potential due to age or longer symptom duration, muscle atrophy, and fatty infiltration. The indications for surgery following conservative treatment are becoming more defined, and an outline regarding what scenarios warrant a transition from an initial conservative treatment plan has been developed. The developing benefits of using mesenchymal stem cells (MSCs) and other biologics have the potential to be disruptive to current treatment protocols in the approaches to healing rotator cuff tears (RCTs). With improved imaging modalities, diagnostic accuracy, and sensitivity, practitioners of the future will hopefully be able to intervene earlier in the disease pathogenesis cycle.

Keywords: natural history, physiotherapy, risk, rotator cuff, biologics

1. Introduction

Rotator cuff disease is prevalent in the general population, accounting for 10% of all shoulder pain and resulting in major shoulder disability. Despite the large prevalence of rotator cuff tears (RCTs), there is still limited information concerning the natural history and treatment approaches for the disorder. An RCT may initially present as a partial-thickness tear (PTT) that progresses to a full-thickness tear (FTT) in the seventh decade of life [1]. Currently, there are no comprehensive British National Institute of Clinical Excellence (NICE) guidelines and European guidelines on the management of RCTs in general, and conclusions made by the American Academy of Orthopaedic Surgeons (AAOS) show weak evidence. Through understanding the natural history of RCTs, the progression from PTT to FTTs, and the different factors that influence progression such as age and comorbidities that influence progression, we can better advise our patients regarding optimum therapy. Such therapies include rehabilitation, physiotherapy, systemic medications and progression to surgical intervention. Although studies regarding physical therapy and surgical interventions show success in the recovery process, it has become increasingly clear that some biologics may augment the healing of tendon to bone when used as a primary treatment or as an adjunct to surgical procedures [2]. However, there are risks of conservative management, and it is important to identify the indications for transition from conservative to surgical management and appreciate patient satisfaction indices. To do so, the authors performed a critical review of the most recent evidence, providing an overview of the best evidence-based management for complete RCTs.

2. Natural history

For appropriate management of RCTs, it is imperative to appreciate the stages of progression of PTTs to FTTs and the contributing factors that lead to symptoms. A thorough patient history includes age, occupation, activities, hand dominance, history of trauma, time since onset of symptoms, history of smoking, diabetes mellitus and patient's expectations. A clinical examination is then supplemented with imaging studies, in particular ultrasound and magnetic resonance imaging (MRI), to further identify the location, size, thickness, retraction of RCTs and any other shoulder pathology such as long head of biceps tendonitis, labral tears, glenohumeral chondrosis, and muscle atrophy.

It is thought that older patients, patients with diabetes mellitus and osteoporosis and smokers will have a less successful repair of a complete tear [3]; however, there is no strong evidence for this. Chronic tears may have poor healing due to associated surrounding fatty infiltration and muscle atrophy [4]. An elderly patient with limited activities may be able to manage activities of daily living with a full-thickness RCT. In contrast, an active young patient may require surgery, even with a small complete RCT.

2.1. Traumatic vs. atraumatic tears

From the patient history, we can establish whether the RCT is a traumatic or degenerative one. Studies by Hantes et al. [5] and Petersen et al. [6] advocate early surgical treatment of complete traumatic RCTs, regardless of size and patient age, to avoid further RCT progression, with subsequent degenerative changes, fatty infiltration of surrounding muscle and cuff retraction. Early surgery should be performed to obtain the best functional results. Atraumatic (degenerative) tears usually occur in elderly patients with larger tears, retracted rotator cuff tendons, poor surrounding tissue and fatty infiltration. In addition, they are likely to have fewer demands from their shoulder. Therefore, surgery may provide a less favourable outcome, and treatment may be best managed conservatively.

2.2. Partial to full-thickness tears

PTTs can be bursal-sided or articular-sided tears. Over the course of time, PTTs enlarge and propagate into FTTs, developing distinct chronic pathological changes due to muscle retraction, fatty infiltration and muscle atrophy. These changes lead to a reduction in tendon elasticity and viability. Although PTT to FTTs are described as a continuum in the literature, these tears can occur without following this natural history path. In its end-state, the glenohumeral joint experiences a series of degenerative alterations known as cuff tear arthropathy.

Maman et al. [7] reported that, based on MRI imaging over an 18-month period for 59 patients, 52% of FTTs will increase in size and were substantially less stable than PTTs. Each shoulder underwent a baseline MRI, and a repeat imaging performed at a minimum interval of 6 months. Progression of tear size was found in 48% of the tears that were followed for at least 18 months compared with just 19% of those followed for less than 18 months. This contrasts with a study by Fucentese et al. [8], who reported seemingly contradictory findings in their report of 24 patients refusing operative treatment for full-thickness supraspinatus tears. They used magnetic resonance arthrography (MRA) as their initial imaging modality and MR without arthrography for their follow-up imaging and reported no increase in the mean size of the RCTs 3.5 years after the initial MRA.

2.3. Small vs. large full-thickness tears

The risk of tear enlargement is greater for shoulders with more advanced tears and is associated with a greater risk of cuff muscle degenerative changes. This group reported that tear enlargement is also associated with greater risk of pain development across all tear types (50% for FTTs) [9].

The same study by Fucentese et al. [8] concludes that small isolated FTTs of the supraspinatus in patients under the age of 65 do not necessarily progress over time. Yamaguchi et al. [10] reported no increase in tear size over 5 years in 23 patients evaluated by ultrasound. This contrasts with a larger case series of 51 patients by Safran et al. [11] which reports that FTTs tend to increase in size in approximately half of patients aged 60 years or younger.

2.4. Demographics

2.4.1. Age

Advancing age has been considered the most important prognostic factor for surgical outcome. Gumina et al. [12] reported that patients older than 60 years of age were twice as likely to develop a tear that was likely to progress to full-thickness and larger tears (54% of tears in patients older than 60 years showed such progression compared to only 17% of tears in those younger than 60 years). A cohort of patients younger than 60 years who were treated non-operatively for FTTs was found to have a higher rate of tear progression than older patients. Of the 61 tears, 49% increased in size according to the findings of ultrasound imaging [11].

2.4.2. Sex

It has generally been reported that there are comparable incidence and characteristics of RCTs in both males and females [12], although only one study by Abate et al. [13] that specifically assessed menopausal women suggested that these women had an increased prevalence of asymptomatic FTT in the postmenopausal period.

2.4.3. Comorbidities

Patient factors such as diabetes mellitus, cigarette smoking and osteoporosis have been suggested to negatively affect the clinical outcomes and healing of RCTs [3, 14].

2.4.4. Hand dominance

There is no clear evidence to associate hand dominance with the development of RCTs [15]; however, one study demonstrated that in the dominant shoulders of 150 veteran competitive tennis players, there were more frequent RCTs, suggesting an association of high-energy activity [16].

2.4.5. Contralateral shoulder

Multiple authors have reported that those who have an established RCT, regardless whether partial or full-thickness and size, are at an increased risk of developing a contralateral RCT [17, 18]. Yamaguchi et al. [10] estimated the prevalence of full-thickness bilateral RCTs at 35%, increasing to as high as 50% in those over the age of 60 years.

2.4.6. Smoking

It is well recognised that smoking reduces microvascular perfusion, possibly reducing rotator cuff tendon vascular perfusion and healing [19]. Baumgarten et al. [20] conducted a study of 375 patients with RCTs confirmed by ultrasound (of all patients presenting with shoulder pain in general, of all demographics and characteristics). Of these 375 patients, 232 (62%) were smokers with a mean 23.4 years of smoking 1.25 packs per day and 30.1 mean pack-years. This is confirmed by the systematic review by Bishop et al. [21] in which increased rates and sizes of rotator cuff degeneration and symptomatic RCTs were seen in smokers, which could consequently increased the number of surgical procedures in these patients. However, there is no case control in these studies, and therefore no strong dose- and time-dependent association between smoking and the development of RCTs could be established.

2.4.7. Family history

There is limited evidence regarding the genetic predisposition and hereditary component for RCTs; however, a study examining the genealogical database in Utah, USA by Tashjian et al. [22] a population-based controlled study of 3091 patients, with a subgroup analysis of 652 patients diagnosed before 40 years of age, showed a significant association between individuals with rotator cuff disease in close and distant relations (reportedly up to third cousin relations). This study was included in the systematic review conducted by Dabija et al. [23], which includes the study by Harvie et al. [24], concluding that siblings of patients diagnosed with RCTs were twice as likely to develop complete RCTs. In addition, they identified single-nucleotide polymorphisms (SNPs) associated with RCTs, indicating the future risk for development of RCTs to enable prophylactic rehabilitation techniques and to avoid the development of symptomatic RCTs [23].

2.4.8. Posture

The relationship between posture and shoulder pathology is still under investigation. For example, Gumina et al. [25] found a reduced subacromial space in 47 patients over the age of 60 years with hyperkyphosis, as compared to a control group. Yamamoto et al. [26] observed RCTs in 65.8% of patients with kyphotic-lordotic postures, 54.3% of patients with flat-back postures, and 48.9% with sway-back postures, whereas only 2.9% of patients with ideal alignment had symptomatic or asymptomatic RCTs. It is hypothesised that the reduced subacromial space is due to less posterior tilting and dyskinesis of the scapula, resulting in extrinsic impingement.

2.4.9. Mental health

Cho et al. [27] demonstrated that as many as 82% of patients with chronic shoulder pain had sleep disturbance and that rates of depression were significantly increased in patients with more than 3 months of shoulder pain. Educational level, employment status, pain levels and patient perception of percentage of shoulder normalcy were most predictive of emotional health in patients with complete RCTs [28].

2.4.10. Symptoms and pain

There is disagreement in the literature regarding the correlation between tear size and pain. These studies tend to be cross-sectional as opposed to prospective observational studies [11]. For example, in a prospective study of 50 patients, Moosmayer et al. [29] reported that 40% of asymptomatic RCTs became symptomatic and anatomically deteriorated, and that an increase in tear size and a decrease in muscle quality correlated with the development of symptoms. Mall et al. [30] who compared asymptomatic and symptomatic RCTs, determined that many with asymptomatic FTTs will develop symptoms with time and that pain development is associated with an increase in tear size and deterioration of shoulder function and active range of motion (ROM). In the study, this was primarily seen with larger tears and required significant time for progression to occur and for glenohumeral and scapular mechanical dysfunction to become apparent. There is therefore the concern that through conservative management of tears, these tears may progress to become more painful. This is supported by the study by Yamaguchi et al. [10] a report of 45 patients, in which 23 (51%) patients became symptomatic at a mean of 2.8 years; however, just 9 of the 23 (39%) demonstrated tear progression; hence, this could mean that over time symptoms can be progressive and not necessarily due to tear size or progression.

Through multiple observational and cross-sectional studies on more than 400 patients with atraumatic, FTTs, the multicenter orthopaedic outcomes network (MOON) Shoulder Group have found that pain and duration of symptoms are not strongly associated with the severity of RCTs [31, 32]. This is supported by a recent cross-sectional study by Curry et al. [33], which found that in patients with RCTs undergoing operative and non-operative treatment, pain and functional status were not associated with tear size and thickness, fatty infiltration, and muscle atrophy.

2.4.11. Radiographic changes

There are studies following the progression of both asymptomatic and symptomatic tears, and most these studies conclude that there is a risk of tear progression according to ultrasound or MRI findings, regardless of whether they are partial or complete RCTs. However, the progression of these tears may not necessarily contribute to increase in symptoms [10]. One ultrasound investigation of 411 patients found the overall prevalence of asymptomatic FTTs to be 13% in patients over age 50 years, and 51% in subjects over 80 years of age [15]. Safran et al. [11] reported that 5 of 61 (8%) FTTs evaluated with ultrasound decreased in size over a 2-year follow-up period.

A recent study by Yang-Soo et al. [34] found that 28 of 34 patients (82.4%) with symptomatic FTTs and 23 of 88 patients (26.1%) with symptomatic PTTs had tears that increased in size over a follow-up period of 6 months to 8 years. The clinical relevance of these observations is that FTTs treated conservatively should be monitored more carefully than PTTs for progression. However, some study limitations should be noted: patients included were those who had refused surgery (allocation bias). In addition, assessor bias due to the reporting of outcomes was a factor; however, the musculoskeletal radiologist reporting the MR images was blind to the clinical data.

This study was supported by another previously described comparison study of 59 shoulders in 54 patients with 33 FTTs, 26 PTTs and 4 combined tears on MRI [7]. Seventeen of 33 (52%) FTTs and 2 of 26 PTTs progressed in size. Factors that were associated with the progression of RCTs were age greater than 60 years, FFTs and fatty infiltration of muscle.

Therefore, RCTs do not always progress, with FTTs demonstrating a higher rate of enlargement in time than PTTs.

3. Effectiveness of physiotherapy rehabilitation

The role of physiotherapy as a form conservative treatment for complete RCTs to improve pain, function, and reduce disability has long been debated. Recently, there have been some studies that have compared the effectiveness of physiotherapy vs. surgical intervention for RCTs.

One systematic review assessed the effectiveness of surgery vs. conservative management of RCTs [35]. It concluded that the three randomised controlled trials that were included in this review showed no statistical or clinically significant difference in the patients' clinical outcomes. One of the limiting factors identified were that two of the studies had a 1-year follow-up in comparison to Moosmayer et al.'s [36] 5-year follow-up. It is therefore difficult to conclude whether the conservative management of the RCTs in the studies was more progressive, or if the surgical repairs failed and the shoulders become symptomatic again. In addition, the systematic review concluded that there were only three trials with adequately varied methods and appropriate inclusion criteria for the review, making it difficult to make a comparison on the overall outcome. This is also supported by a systematic review by Seida [37], who concluded that there was insufficient evidence to support conservative over surgical treatment and vice versa for the management of RCTs and suggested that further studies were required and standardised methods and inclusion criteria were warranted.

The first randomised controlled trial by Moosmayer et al. [36] after 5 years showed no significance between surgery and physiotherapy, as the mean difference in the Constant-Murley Score (CMS) was only 5, which is deemed less than that considered a clinically relevant score of 10.4 [38]. This study also had traumatic tears in the conservative group, which may have influenced the results as previous research has suggested that early surgical intervention is recommended for younger patients with traumatic tears and severe functional deficit to avoid delays in tendon healing or prevent healing beyond repair [39]. The sample size was small in this study; therefore, it is difficult to make a conclusion on the effect of having the two subgroups over the results in this study. In this study, nine patients failed physiotherapy and switched to tendon repair in small and medium tears. Rotator cuff repairs may be recommended to prevent delay in progression of muscle atrophy and tendon retraction beyond the point of tendon healing if physiotherapy failed, which is more likely in the younger patient population with acute tears than in the older population who are more likely to present with degenerative FTTs [40, 41]. This is further supported by an algorithm on the management of RCTs by Tashijan [42] according to size, nature of the tear, and age of the patient; however, there is not enough high-quality evidence to support this. Further studies comparing interventions for traumatic and atraumatic complete tears as well as age groups would be required to decide initial treatment. In addition, further research on how long conservative management should be continued before resorting to surgical intervention would be required. This finding has also been discussed by Abdulwahab et al. [43], who concluded that timing to the end of conservative treatment is unknown, but likely is indicated when a patient demonstrates increased weakness and loss of function not recoverable by physiotherapy.

Another randomised controlled trial by Heerspink et al. [44] was a small study of only 56 patients that showed no statistical or clinically significant difference. The CMS was 10.1 between surgery and physiotherapy. The patients in this study were atraumatic, which may have made the study more generalised compared to Moosmayer's randomised controlled trial [36]. There were more patients with a larger tear in the conservative treatment group, which could have created bias in the results of this study despite the random allocation. Further research on surgical intervention compared to physiotherapy for complete tears as a separate entity from partial tears are needed. In addition, high-quality studies in which comparisons between different conservative interventions and surgical treatment are made to determine the optimal conservative management for RCTs are necessary.

The present study also had a high incidence (73%) of re-tears in the surgical repair group at 1-year follow-up. However, tear progression or failed rotator cuff repair may not be indicative of why the patients have more pain and less function, as studies have shown that large tears can be asymptomatic [45, 46]. This uncertainty in the extent of RCTs in relation to the patient's clinical presentation may not be an accurate representation of the outcome of the patient's pain and function post intervention in this study. The best pain and functional outcomes in this study were observed in surgical patients with an intact rotator cuff repair at the final follow-up, but the numbers to treat for successful rotator cuff repair would be high in this case considering the 73% of failed repairs that reported slightly less favourable outcome than the conservative approach. The insignificant difference in the outcome of this study demonstrates that physiotherapy may possibly be considered as an intervention due to it being less expensive than surgery as reported in this article. However, longer duration of follow-ups in this study would be beneficial to determine the outcome of both interventions in relation to MRI findings, pain, function and economic impact.

Kukkonen et al. [47] concluded in their 1-year follow-up study that there was no statistical significance between rotator cuff repair with acromioplasty and physiotherapy, or physiotherapy alone. There was only a difference in patient satisfaction scores in the first 3 and 6 months, where the two groups without repair reported higher patient satisfaction than the repair group. This may be due to the postoperative restrictions for the surgery group, leading to more dissatisfaction in this group. However, the overall outcome was the same by the 1-year follow-up

Overall, the three studies showed low risk of bias that cannot completely be avoided because of the nature of interventions. Despite the conservative and surgical interventions in all three trials being standardised with the same treatment aims, the patients' irritability and severity of their symptoms and the effect on their daily function varied the intensity, dosage, and duration of treatment. This variation made it difficult to compare conservative and surgical approaches for the management of RCTs. The treatment strategies and aims among all three trials for physiotherapy were similar in that all three randomised controlled trials focused on initiating static and dynamic glenohumeral movement, scapulohumeral movement, and stabilisation, and increasing the level of progression from 6 to 12 weeks.

3.1. Physiotherapy treatment techniques

There is some debate on the optimal conservative treatment and rehabilitation approach for RCTs and its role in improving the symptoms associated with an RCT.

Ainsworth et al. [48] conducted a systematic review of exercise therapy for the conservative management of RCTs. This review could not find any high-quality trials and found only 10 observational studies and 2 case studies. The primary conclusion of this review was that physiotherapy may have some benefit; however, the method of distinguishing the extent of the patient's pain in relation to the tear as well as the level of exercise in terms of intensity and dosage are still unclear due to the poor quality of the trials.

The review also concluded that the size of the tear is not as important as the presence of pain in the patient. This is supported by the findings discussed previously with the current research and MRI scans in relation to the patient's clinical symptoms. It also highlighted that RCT repairs appear to be less successful in the elderly, and the review lean more towards conservative management as a first line of treatment. This idea is also supported by the Tashjian algorithm [42] and Levy [49], who further explain that due to older patients being more likely to have multiple comorbidities, RCTs should be managed conservatively.

The present study acknowledged that until there is more understanding of how some patients with FTTs can have a spectrum of symptoms from minimum to severe, it will be difficult to establish an optimal treatment and rehabilitation program for RCTs.

There are differences in opinion on the focus of rehabilitation between anterior deltoid retraining or working on the humeral head depressors to rehabilitate shoulder elevation in abduction only [50]. The anterior deltoid training is supported by Levy et al. [49] and by Ainsworth [51] on the basis of the biomechanics of how the anterior deltoid works. The anterior deltoid was believed to act as a humeral head elevator, but a study by Gagey and Hue [52] concluded that the deltoid functions to prevent upward migration of the humeral head. This theory is supported in present clinical practice of using the Torbay exercise program, which is proposed in the aforementioned studies. In the Levy et al. study [49] instructions were to exercise 3–5 times per day for the first 6 weeks, with the patient supine for the exercises, and progressing to an incline, and then standing. This study found that this technique would be beneficial for older patients with atraumatic, massive tears. However, this study was not compared with another intervention; therefore, there was no randomised allocation, and the lack of quality and a small study group of 17 patients made it difficult to form a significant conclusion.

Ainsworth et al.'s [48] prospective randomised controlled study had 60 patients over the course of 1 year. The intervention group consisted of anterior deltoid training as well as other treatment modalities such as functional exercises, proprioception and stretching. It is therefore difficult to establish which specific treatment modality had an impact on improving patient pain and function compared to the control group, whose treatment consisted of ultrasound, advice, and steroid injections, if required. The SF-36 score showed statistical significance in the intervention group over the control group at 3 and 6 months, but there were no differences by 12 months. Despite these improvements in functional and pain scores, further studies with standardised treatment interventions and larger numbers of patients over a longer period are needed to support the use of anterior deltoid training.

This study also highlighted the role of education in altering the patient's perception of pain and therefore reduce pain and disability, which is also supported in previous studies [53, 54]. It is believed that advice and education alone allow the patient to use the shoulder, by reducing their fears of causing more harm. This may have contributed to why the control group had no statistical difference from the intervention group. Despite these findings, physiotherapy with this specific anterior deltoid exercise program is deemed to be beneficial because it allows patients to return to their activities of daily living (ADLs) earlier, which could impact aspects such as reducing time away from work and the risk of depression, and improving quality of life (which are associated with poor outcome). Future studies should further investigate this exercise program. Kuhn et al. [55] conducted a multi-centre prospective cohort study of 381 patients who underwent physiotherapy over a 12-week period with a 2-year follow-up. The patients' compliance diaries showed a variation in programs from no therapy to supervision and home, home only, and supervision only. If after 6 weeks the patients were no longer in pain and/or the pain was not affecting their ADLs, then conservative management was successful. Only 9% of patients had surgery after 6 weeks, and a total of 15% of patients had surgery in the first 12 months. After this time, it is deemed that the patient is unlikely to have surgery for RCT. This study was performed only on atraumatic patients only; thus, it is not a reflection of acute traumatic tears. The treatment strategies for these patients were primarily focused on exercise therapy, manual therapy, and heat and cold therapy. However, there were no comparison intervention groups to establish which treatment modality was superior to another, and the therapist could tailor the therapy to the patient's individual presentation, making it difficult to form a conclusion on the most effective aspect of the therapy program. Edwards et al. [56] conducted a review of the current treatment strategies during rehabilitation and concluded the use of anterior deltoid training allows adequate shoulder elevation without upward migration of the humeral head. In this review, the authors also noted the role of the teres minor during external rotation with infraspinatus tears as part of allowing the greater tuberosity of the humerus to clear the acromion during shoulder elevation. Studies that have been researched currently show a general trend of 10–15 repetitions twice a day; however, further research to justify using the prescription recommended for this specific type of training is warranted.

It appears that the nature of the studies that have been reviewed do not always focus on complete RCTs, which is due to the lack of available evidence on the management of complete RCTs. Therefore, the conclusions in this review are limited. More studies focusing on the surgical and conservative management of complete RCTs need to be completed to delve further into the optimal management of this pathology.

4. Systemic medications

It is unclear if there is a true inflammatory element to rotator cuff tendinopathy and whether non-steroidal anti-inflammatory drugs (NSAIDs) will address this pathophysiology [57]. Currently, no trial or study has been conducted for evaluating NSAIDs as an oral preparation or topically, or other analgesics specifically, for efficacy in the treatment of complete RCTs. Only investigations for shoulder pain in general have been conducted [43]. One meta-analysis of 12 studies concludes that oral NSAIDs can lead to a reduction in pain in individuals with rotator cuff tendinopathy, but there are gastrointestinal or cardiovascular-associated risks [58].

5. Injections

The concept of using injections for the treatment of RCTs is not new to the field of orthopaedic surgery, as the practice of using injections such as corticosteroids (CS) and sodium hyaluronate (HA) is common in many practices. CS and HA are both injectable pharmaceutical agents that can be used to decrease pain and stiffness, and they have demonstrated significant impact on improving quality of life for patients with RCTs.

A 2015 in vitro study found that CS injections decreased cell proliferation in rotator cuff tendons, and the resulting strength of these tendons decreased as compared to the strength after HA injections [59]. The same study also conducted an experiment on the effects of CS and HA injections in rats. Like the in vitro study, the animal study found apoptosis in rotator cuff tendons, inhibition of cell proliferation, a delay in tendon healing, and decreased biomechanical strength in CS subjects [59].

Clinical application of these agents is highlighted by a study conducted in 2001, in which 40% of a group with RCTs that received HA injections were satisfied with the durable effects produced at 24-weeks follow-up [60]. In addition, 35% of the group that received CS injections expressed satisfaction over a 5-week period with the injections [60]. Moreover, another study found statistically significant pain relief in groups with HA injections as compared to the control group [61]. In another study, a combination of HA injections and rehabilitation programs led to an improvement of mobility in elderly patients [62]. When using CS injections, no difference was found in groups with different frequencies of injections [63].

6. Biologics

6.1. Basic science

Biologics are similar to the aforementioned injections, as they are injected into the RCT zone to assist in regeneration of the tendons. Biologics are specific proteins and cells that are obtained from the patient; therefore, they are personalised for the individual [64].

Biological injections can include platelet-rich plasma (PRP), which is prepared from a patient's blood by concentrating thrombocytes, usually a multiple of the normal circulating concentration. This injection is produced through standardised preparations: blood is drawn from the patient and spun in a centrifuge to separate the parts of the blood, and the highly concentrated plasma is re-administered to the patient in the affected area [65]. The idea of PRP follows simple scientific logic as the platelets are the body's primary way of reaching structural defects and injuries through proteins, cytokines, and growth factors that stimulate healing. Once platelets reach the specific site, they release different growth hormones that trigger natural and regenerative healing processes [66]. PRP has been known to stimulate both the response of mesenchymal stem cells (MSCs) to the local area through growth factors such as platelet-derived growth factor (PDGF), fibroblast growth factor and vascular endothelial growth factor

(VEGF) and stimulate tendon stem cells to differentiate into tenocytes when certain growth factors are released, which promotes healing of the rotator cuff [67, 68]. Furthermore, PRP can also assist in the proliferation of muscle cells [69], promoting inflammation [70], and the use of adhesion molecules to repair the torn tendon [71]. The proliferation of muscle cells allows for an increased number of fibroblasts and myotubes, thereby decreasing the overall time of recovery and increasing the strength of the rotator cuff [69]. Non-growth factors released from platelets such as serotonin, histamine, dopamine, calcium and adenosine aid in inflammation proliferation [70]. Finally, adhesion molecules such as fibronectin, fibrin and vitronectin can be delivered in a clot [71].

MSCs can be found in a variety of locations throughout the human body, but are most commonly found around vascular tissue, bone marrow, and fat [72]. MSCs are derived from pericytes that detach from the blood vessels and become activated MSCs [72]. These stem cells, like many other stem cells, can proliferate and eventually differentiate into fully functional osteocytes, adipocytes, and fibroblasts or remain as activated MSCs [73]. MSCs can be both immunomodulatory and trophic, which aid in regeneration. The cells can act as an auto-immune response to combat pathogens that infect the ruptured tissue [74]. Further, MSCs inhibit both apoptosis (cell death) and scar formation while stimulating angiogenesis and mitosis (through the secretion of mitogens) [64]. Because of the many functions of MSCs, the activation of MSCs is critical in the healing process. These activated MSC cells provide the damaged part with necessary chemicals to heal itself more quickly.

6.2. Laboratory investigation

An in vitro study found that PRP stimulated cell proliferation and the synthesis of tenocytes in RCTs [75]. In an experiment in which rats were treated for RCT, the group given the PRP treatment demonstrated better collagen linear alignment. Furthermore, the research team found positive effects when administering the PRP injections 3 weeks after the initial surgery [76].

6.3. Clinical investigation

A clinical trial in 2012 found reduced pain and positive effects in the healing process of RCTs [77]. These clinical trials demonstrate the effect PRP has in stimulating the already present natural healing process.

A commonly used source for regenerative injection therapy (RIT) is bone marrow aspirate that is centrifuged to form a concentrate. Bone marrow aspirate concentrate (BMAC) can possess a number of different stem or progenitor cells that can aid in the body's natural self-regenerative processes [78]. BMAC can be used as a regenerative injection therapy for various injuries and primary conditions, as well as be used during surgery. One study compared BMAC augmented surgery vs. arthroscopic repair alone. Of the 45 patients augmented with BMAC, 100% of patients were healed 6 months after surgery compared to 67% of the 45 control patients. At 10-year follow-up found that 87% of patients in the BMAC group compared with 44% of control patients were healed [79].

7. Risks of conservative treatment in managing a rotator cuff tear

Non-operative treatment has been recommended as an initial treatment for patients with rotator cuff pathology ranging from tendinopathy to partial and even complete RCTs [80]. Although several reviews and studies have demonstrated the effectiveness of non-operative treatment in RCTs, as previously described, there are concerns regarding the risks of conservative treatment as well. The overall goal of conservative management is to diminish pain, increase ROM and strength, and to ultimately decrease the functional limitations of the patient [81]. There appears to be some consensus that a conservative treatment program is a reasonable approach within the first 6–12 weeks in patients with non-traumatic tears under the age of 60 years. If the patient does not respond within the initial 4–6 weeks, then it can be an indicator for transition to surgical treatment. Edwards et al. [56] has demonstrated that if the patient does respond well, the conservative treatment will be effective for up to 2 years. Tanaka et al. [81] reviewed the literature and noted that conservative treatment is an effective method for the treatment of RCTs, with success rates ranging from 33 to 88%. The large variability appears to be dependent on the method of treatment chosen, as well as the observations and monitoring that occurs in between the pre-established patient follow-up dates. Although effective, the benefits of non-operative treatment have also been accompanied by progression of the tear, muscle atrophy, fatty infiltration, worse surgical outcomes and increased pain and symptoms.

Tempelhof et al. [15] studied asymptomatic RCTs longitudinally to improve the understanding of the risks of tear progression and pain development over time. The study followed patients for a median of 5.1 years, following the identification of the asymptomatic degenerative tear. They observed that tear enlargement occurred in a time-dependent manner with greater risks of enlargement relative to larger and more severe tears. This was observed in 110 of 224 patients (~49%) over an average span of 2.8 years. FTTs were 1.5–4 times more likely to enlarge than PTTs. In addition to the risk of tear progression, the transition from an asymptomatic tear to a symptomatic tear was observed due to the development of new pain, and the median time until pain developed was roughly 2.6 years. The development of new pain occurred in 46% of the patients, and the occurrence of symptoms correlated with an average enlargement rate of 63%, whereas those who remained asymptomatic had a 38% increase in the size of their tears.

These results demonstrate the long-term potential for an FTT to increase in size over several years, which is in agreement with Hsu and Keener [82], who thought that the risks of tear progression and muscle atrophy are present early on, but the rate of progression is slow enough to allow adequate time to attempt conservative treatment [82]. They developed a stratification of the several treatment options in which the patients were categorised and recommended a treatment option based on their natural history and pathology. The system established by Hsu and Keener [82] contained three groups in which the risks of non-operative treatment varied and the potential benefits of surgery were optimised. The groups were assigned according to the symptoms presented at the time of the patient interview. In group I, early operative repair was recommended for acute tears, while those in group

II were initially treated conservatively and, if they did not respond, they were transitioned to surgical treatment. Furthermore, group III was concerned with maximising conservative treatment, where the healing of the patient's RCT was unlikely. This group typically included patients over the age of 65, with chronic tears and FTT. Patients in the group were shown to have retracted tendons and advanced muscle degeneration. The goal of conservative treatment was to improve the overall functioning level of the patient. This study demonstrated that although these variables improved, there was also a 50% chance of tear progression within 5 years, especially in the FTT [82].

Several other studies of asymptomatic tears followed by either an ultrasound or a MRI have been reported in the literature [2, 15, 83, 84]. Maman et al. [7] described age as a large determinant of progression, with 54% of the tears in the patients over 60 years of age demonstrating progression, in comparison to 17% of tears in subjects under the age of 60 years. Safran et al. [11] found that FTTs had a higher rate of progression in younger patients, with 49% of the tears increasing in size under ultrasound.

Tear progression as well as muscle atrophy and fatty infiltration have been directly associated with pain. In a study conducted by Moosmayer et al. [85], these three variables were found to correlate with the presence of symptoms in comparison to an asymptomatic group. The authors compared non-operative to operative treatment for smaller tears of 3 cm in size, and found a progression in tear size and structural deterioration over time, which resulted in the recurrence of symptoms and functional depreciation over time. In the cases in which the patients were asymptomatic, they found that progression of the tear was directly related with the development of pain [30].

In contrast to these studies, Fucentese et al. [8] found that after a follow-up period of 3.5 years following non-operative treatment, there was no increase in the average tear size and only 25% of the initial tears demonstrated progression. An issue with this study is that the average initial tear size was small, averaging 1.6 cm. This further supports the notion that the likelihood of progression is dependent on the initial size of the tear, with larger tears more likely to develop progression.

8. Surgical indications for a transition from non-operative treatment

Throughout the literature, it has been observed that the presence of certain independent "risk factors" may also serve as indicators for the physician to transfer the patient from non-operative management to operative treatment. Beyond the risks and concerns involved with the non-operative treatment option, there are also independent factors that serve as direct indicators to opt for operative treatment. These factors include the patient's demographics, the mechanism of injury, the degree of severity and depth of the tear, the duration of symptoms and the patient's expectations about whether operative or non-operative treatments are effective. Several studies [2, 82, 86] have shown that patient expectations are potentially one of the strongest indicators when deciding how to treat a patient. Dunn et al. [87] and Fucentese et al. [8] demonstrated a direct correlation between the expectations of the patient and the results of conservative treatment.

The demographics of a patient have also been shown to directly correspond with a transition in treatment. The strongest of these include the patient's age, body mass index (BMI) score, and socioeconomic status. Interestingly, patients with a higher BMI score were shown to be more likely to adopt a nonsurgical option, where those with a lower BMI opted for surgical treatment [88].

Regarding age, patients under the age of 60 years are thought to have better outcomes with operative treatment, because of significant risks of irreversible changes with non-operative treatment and a high likelihood of healing if a repair was performed. It has been generally recommended that surgical repair be performed instead of an initial conservative treatment in active patients with acute tears following trauma [4]. Early operative treatment appears to be warranted in this case and in the case of poor function for the achievement of maximal return of shoulder function. The importance of the timing following the initial patient interview is critical and dependent on the factors associated with the tear as well as how long the tear has been present. In a systematic review, Lazarides et al. [40] reported that the RCTs present in patients younger than age 40 years are more commonly FTTs and of traumatic origin. These patients typically respond well to surgery in terms of pain relief due to the good tendon and muscle quality at the time of the repair. The definition of "early" repair is often unclear.

Bjornsson et al. [89] determined that there was no difference in tendon healing, pain, shoulder elevation, or functional outcomes when an acute tear was fixed within the first 3 months of injury compared to within the first 3 weeks. However, if symptoms have persisted for longer than a year, and functional impairment was observed, the expectation for a successful surgical approach is worse in patients with FTTs [56]. Patients over the age of 60 years were twice as likely to develop a tear that was larger than those under 60 years. With each decade after 60, the odds of tear enlargement increased 2.69-fold [90].

Importantly, the mechanism of injury plays a significant role in decision-making for operative treatment. Schmidt and Morrey [91] described a measurement of the "appropriateness" of the various treatment options available to assist in RCT treatment, which are dependent on the associated benefits and risks of each method. The scale is referred to as the appropriate use criteria (AUC), and it was developed by a voting panel composed of mostly orthopaedic surgeons. This panel determined the 'appropriateness' level of a treatment based on the current literature. The AUC determined that a treatment was deemed 'appropriate' if the benefits outweighed the risks, 'may be appropriate' if the difference was null, and 'rarely Appropriate' when the risks outweighed the benefits. A large indicator favouring non-operative treatment included the initial response a patient exhibited during their initial trial of conservative treatment. If there was a positive response noted by the patient, then they would continue with non-operative treatment. Conversely, if the initial trial of conservative treatment was ineffective, then operative treatment would be recommended. The indications for surgery were 'may be appropriate' in the instances in which the patient responded positively to the conservative management, were healthy before the injury, were experiencing moderate-to-severe pain, as well as in those who were not responsive to non-operative care methods. The duration of time given to determine whether a conservative treatment option is successful is typically 12 weeks. Beyond this time, there was a concern regarding the risk of tear progression. In addition, the authors showed that in patients with a higher level of pain, they were more likely to recommend surgery.

If surgery is needed in case of failed conservative treatment, chances for tendon healing are much lower after the age of 60 years [92]. In selected cases, surgery may be limited to a simple arthroscopic biceps tenotomy while leaving the cuff unrepaired with good pain relief and shoulder function in the elderly [93]. In other cases, despite older age, repairing the cuff may still be an option with high subjective patient satisfaction rates [94].

9. Patient satisfaction indices

In a study of 20 patients conducted by Baydar et al. [86], 6 months following conservative treatment 55% of the patients reported that they were 'much better' and 45% said they were 'better'. At their 1-year follow-up, 50% rated themselves as 'much better' and 40% rated themselves as 'better'. This trend was also observed at the 3-year follow-up.

Kuhn et al. [55] conducted a study over a 3-month period and found that physiotherapy significantly improved pain, function and ROM. Wirth et al. [95] conducted a similar study of 60 patients, with a 2-year follow-up. On the basis of the American Shoulder and Elbow Surgeons evaluation (ASES) and the UCLA score, they found that the patients showed significant improvements. They noted improved pain ratings, strength, and ROM.

Boorman et al. [96] found 75% of the patients were successfully treated conservatively. They noted that the baseline rotator cuff quality-of-life index (RC-QOL) score was a significant predictor of the outcome. Eighty-nine percent of the patients maintained their 3-month outcome at the 2-year follow-up. Even subjects with increased pain and tear progression were shown to have a significant increase in their functional scores.

10. Discussion

RCTs in general are prevalent within the population of all age groups. FTTs can present acutely following trauma or as a degenerative process. We have examined the associations with genetic influences, comorbidities, and the complex relationship between tear size, symptoms, and pain. Although there is conflicting literature, there appears to be some consensus on the best indicators for choosing to treat a FTT non-operatively. The established physiotherapy techniques include anterior deltoid training to allow adequate shoulder elevation without upward migration of the humeral head, as well as teres minor training to allow the greater tuberosity of the humerus to clear the acromion during shoulder elevation. Patients who will benefit the most from conservative treatment include those over the age of 60 years with a chronic degenerative tear that is unlikely to heal and with low functional demand. In this scenario, the goal is to improve the function and ROM. The risks associated with these tears include the potential of the progression of the tear, a diminished healing potential due to age or longer symptom duration, muscle atrophy, and fatty infiltration. In addition, poor outcomes have been noted in this group with surgical treatment. Moreover, the indications for surgery following conservative treatment are becoming more defined, and an outline regarding what scenarios warrant a transition from an initial conservative treatment plan has been developed. If the patient does not respond well within the first 6–12 weeks of the conservative treatment and is younger than 60 years, has a higher activity level, and has a healthy tendon and muscle environment, then early operative treatment is likely. Overall, the patient satisfaction indices, and in particular functional scores such as the RC-QOL score, have shown a consistent level of satisfaction regarding conservative management in patients followed from 2 years.

Although experiments using injections and biologics to specifically treat RCTs are limited, the literature available is promising in primary treatment, adjunctive care, and to augment surgical procedures. Both CS and HA injections offer modest benefits to the patient in terms of reduced pain and improved function. From an administrative perspective, the injections are practical as they are easily available pharmaceuticals, and are relatively low in prices compared to surgical intervention. These injections have demonstrated effectiveness in ameliorating symptoms following RCT.

The developing benefits of using MSCs, PRP, and other biologics have the potential to be disruptive to current treatment protocols, both conservative as well as surgical, in the approaches to healing RCTs. With improved imaging modalities, diagnostic accuracy, and sensitivity, practitioners of the future will hopefully be able to intervene earlier in the disease pathogenesis cycle. PRP can possibly be an effective method and strategy in the healing process of tendinopathy or PTTs. With standardised preparations and treatment protocols, only a short window of time is required to assess, prepare, and treat patients with this method (less than 30 minutes). The real benefit, although not fully realised at this time, is that PRP follows fundamental biological principles as it releases several growth hormones to stimulate the healing process. PRP also prompts MSC activation, creating a unique regenerative environment that modulates the immune system response and promotes trophic, anti-scarring, and cellular proliferation that in theory further aid the healing process. Regenerative injection therapy provides patients with specific cells and proteins that their body has produced, thus creating a healing environment at the site of injury and/or degeneration. Further studies in the basic science, translation, as well as with high-quality clinical trials are needed to shed further light on this very exciting and potentially game-changing technology.

Author details

Taiceer A. Abdulwahab[1]*, William D. Murrell[2], Frank Z. Jenio[2], Navneet Bhangra[3], Gerard A. Malanga[4], Michael Stafford[4], Nitin B. Jain[5] and Olivier Verborgt[6]

*Address all correspondence to: taiceer.abdulwahab@doctors.org.uk

1 Department of Orthopaedic Surgery, Mediclinic City Hospital, Dubai, United Arab Emirates

2 Sapphire Surgery and Medical Centre, Emirates Hospitals Group, Dubai, United Arab Emirates

3 Mediclinic Mirdif, Dubai, United Arab Emirates

4 Rutgers School of Medicine – New Jersey Medical School, New Jersey, USA

5 Vanderbilt University School of Medicine, Nashville, USA

6 AZ Monica Hospital, Antwerp, Belgium

References

[1] Murrell WD, Anz AW, Badsha H, Bennett WF, Boykin RE, Caplan AI. Regenerative treatments to enhance orthopedic surgical outcome. Physical Medicine and Rehabilitation. 2015;7:S41-S52. DOI: 10.1016/j.pmrj.2015.01.015

[2] Milgrom C, Schaffler M, Gilbert S, van Holsbeeck M. Rotator-cuff changes in asymptomatic adults. The effect of age, hand dominance and gender. Journal of Bone and Joint Surgery (British). 1995;77(2):296-298

[3] Chung SW, Oh JH, Gong HS, Kim JY, Kim SH. Factors affecting rotator cuff healing after arthroscopic repair: Osteoporosis as one of the independent risk factors. The American Journal of Sports Medicine. 2011;39(10):2099-2107

[4] Dwyer T, Razmjou H, Henry P, Gosselin-Fournier S, Holtby R. Association between preoperative magnetic resonance imaging and reparability of large and massive rotator cuff tears. Knee Surgery, Sports Traumatology, Arthroscopy. 2015;23(2):415-422

[5] Hantes ME, Karidakis GK, Vlychou M, et al. A comparison of early versus delayed repair of traumatic rotator cuff tears. Knee Surgery, Sports Traumatology, Arthroscopy. 2011;19:1766-1770

[6] Petersen SA, Murphy TP. The timing of rotator cuff repair for the restoration of function. Journal of Shoulder and Elbow Surgery. 2011;20:62-68

[7] Maman E, Harris C, White L, et al. Outcome of nonoperative treatment of symptomatic rotator cuff tears monitored by magnetic resonance imaging. The Journal of Bone and Joint Surgery. American Volume. 2009;91:1898-1906

[8] Fucentese SF, von Roll AL, Pfirrmann CW, et al. Evolution of non- operatively treated symptomatic isolated full-thickness supraspinatus tears. The Journal of Bone and Joint Surgery. American Volume. 2012;**94**:801-808

[9] Keener JD, Galatz LM, Teefey SA, et al. A prospective evaluation of survivorship of asymptomatic degenerative rotator cuff tears. The Journal of Bone and Joint Surgery. American Volume. 2015;**97**(2):89-98

[10] Yamaguchi K, Tetro AM, Blam O, Evanoff BA, Teefey SA, Middleton WD. Natural history of asymptomatic rotator cuff tears: A longitudinal analysis of asymptomatic tears detected sonographically. Journal of Shoulder and Elbow Surgery. 2001;**10**(3):199-203

[11] Safran O, Schroeder J, Bloom R, Weil Y, Milgrom C. Natural history of nonoperatively treated symptomatic rotator cuff tears in patients 60 years old or younger. The American Journal of Sports Medicine. 2011;**39**(4):710-714

[12] Gumina S, Carbone S, Campagna V, Candela V, Sacchetti FM, Giannicola G. The impact of aging on rotator cuff tear size. Musculoskeletal Surgery. 2013;**97**(Suppl 1): 69-72

[13] Abate M, Schiavone C, Di Carlo L, Salini V. Prevalence of and risk factors for asymptomatic rotator cuff tears in postmenopausal women. Menopause. 2014;**21**:275-280

[14] Clement ND, Hallett A, MacDonald D, Howie C, McBirnie J. Does diabetes affect outcome after arthroscopic repair of the rotator cuff? Journal of Bone and Joint Surgery (British). 2010;**92**(8):1112-1117

[15] Tempelhof S, Rupp S, Seil R. Age-related prevalence of rotator cuff tears in asymptomatic shoulders. Journal of Shoulder and Elbow Surgery. 1999;**8**:296-299

[16] Brasseur JL, Lucidarme O, Tardieu M, Tordeur M, Montalvan B, Parier J, Le Goux P, Gires A, Grenier P. Ultrasonographic rotator cuff changes in veteran tennis players: The effect of hand dominance and comparison with clinical findings. European Radiology. 2004;**14**:857-864

[17] Liem D, Buschmann VE, Schmidt C, Gosheger G, Vogler T, Schulte TL, Balke M. The prevalence of rotator cuff tears: Is the contralateral shoulder at risk? The American Journal of Sports Medicine. 2014;**42**:826-830

[18] Ro KH, Park JH, Lee SH, Song DI, Jeong HJ, Jeong WK. Status of the contralateral rotator cuff in patients undergoing rotator cuff repair. The American Journal of Sports Medicine. 2015;**43**:1091-1098

[19] Carbone S, Gumina S, Arceri V, Campagna V, Fagnani C, Postacchini F. The impact of preoperative smoking habit on rotator cuff tear: Cigarette smoking influences rotator cuff tear sizes. Journal of Shoulder and Elbow Surgery. 2012;21:56-60

[20] Baumgarten KM, Gerlach D, Galatz LM, Teefey SA, Middleton WD, Ditsios K, Yamaguchi K. Cigarette smoking increases the risk for rotator cuff tears. Clinical Orthopaedics and Related Research. 2010;**468**:1534-1541

[21] Bishop JY, SantiagoTorres JE, Rimmke N, Flanigan DC. Smoking predisposes to rotator cuff pathology and shoulder dysfunction: A systematic review. Arthroscopy. 2015;**31**:1598-1605

[22] Tashjian R, Farnham J, Albright F, Teerlink C, Cannon-Albright L. Evidence for an inherited predisposition contributing to the risk for rotator cuff. The Journal of Bone and Joint Surgery. 2009;**91**(5):1136-1142

[23] Dabija D, Gao C, Edwards T, Kuhn J, Jain N. Genetic and familial predisposition to rotator cuff disease: A systematic review. Journal of Shoulder and Elbow Surgery. 2017;**26**(6):1103-1112

[24] Harvie P, Ostlere S, Teh J, Mcnally E, Clipsham K, Burston B, Pollard T, Carr A. Genetic influences in the aetiology of tears of the rotator cuff. The Journal of Bone and Joint Surgery. 2004;**86**(5):696-700

[25] Gumina S, Di Giorgio G, Postacchini F, Postacchini R. Suba cromial space in adult patients with thoracic hyperkyphosis and in healthy volunteers. Chirurgia Degli Organi di Movimento. 2008;**91**:93-96

[26] Yamamoto A, Takagishi K, Kobayashi T, Shitara H, Ichinose T, Takasawa E, Shimoyama D, Osawa T. The impact of faulty posture on rotator cuff tears with and without symptoms. Journal of Shoulder and Elbow Surgery. 2015;24:446-452

[27] Cho CH, Jung SW, Park JY, Song KS, Yu KI. Is shoulder pain for three months or longer correlated with depression, anxiety, and sleep disturbance? Journal of Shoulder and Elbow Surgery. 2013;**22**:222-228

[28] Barlow J, Bishop J, Dunn W, Kuhn J. What factors are predictors of emotional health in patients with full-thickness rotator cuff tears? Journal of Shoulder and Elbow Surgery. 2016;**25**(11):1769-1773

[29] Moosmayer S, Tariq R, Stiris M, et al. The natural history of asymptomatic rotator cuff tears: A three-year follow-up of fifty cases. The Journal of Bone and Joint Surgery. American Volume. 2013;**95**:1249-1255

[30] Mall NA, Kim HM, Keener JD, et al. Symptomatic progression of asymptomatic rotator cuff tears: A prospective study of clinical and sonographic variables. The Journal of Bone and Joint Surgery. American Volume. 2010;**92**:2623-2633

[31] Group MS, Unruh KP, Kuhn JE, et al. The duration of symptoms does not correlate with rotator cuff tear severity or other patient-related features: A cross-sectional study of patients with atraumatic, full-thickness rotator cuff tears. Journal of Shoulder and Elbow Surgery. 2014;**23**:1052-1058

[32] Dunn W, Kuhn J, Sanders R, An Q, Baumgarten K, Bishop J, Brophy R, Carey J, Holloway G, Jones G, Ma C, Marx R, McCarty E, Poddar S, Smith M, Spencer E, Vidal A, Wolf B, Wright R. Symptoms of pain do not correlate with rotator cuff tear severity. The Journal of Bone & Joint Surgery, 2014;**96**(10):793-800

[33] Curry EJ, Matzkin E, Dong Y, Higgins LD, Katz JN, Jain NB. Structural characteristics are not associated with pain and function in rotator cuff tears: The ROW cohort study. Orthopaedic Journal of Sports Medicine. 2015;3(5):1-7

[34] Kim Y, Kim S, Bae S, Lee H, Jee W, Park C. Tear progression of symptomatic full-thickness and partial-thickness rotator cuff tears as measured by repeated MRI. Knee Surgery, Sports Traumatology, Arthroscopy. 2016;25(7):2073-2080

[35] Ryösä A, Laimi K, Äärimaa V, Lehtimäki K, Kukkonen J, Saltychev M. Surgery or conservative treatment for rotator cuff tear: A meta-analysis. Disability and Rehabilitation. 2016;39(14):1357-1363

[36] Moosmayer S, Lund G, Seljom US, Haldorsen B, Svege IC, Hennig T, et al. Tendon repair compared with physiotherapy in the treatment of rotator cuff tears. The Journal of Bone and Joint Surgery. American Volume. 2014;96:1504-1514. DOI: 10.2106/jbjs.m.01393

[37] Seida JC, Jennifer C. Systematic review: Nonoperative and operative treatments for rotator cuff tears. Annals of Internal Medicine. 2010;153(4):246

[38] Kukkonen J, Kauko T, Vahlberg Hlberg T, Joukainen A, Aarimaa V. Investigating minimal clinical importance difference for Constant Score in patients undergoing rotator cuff surgery. Journal of Shoulder and Elbow Surgery. 2013 Dec;22(12):1650-1655

[39] Habermeyer P, Schuller U, Wiedemann E. The intra-articular pressure of the shoulder: An experimental study on the role of the glenoid labrum in stabilizing the joint. Arthroscopy: The Journal of Arthroscopic & Related Surgery. 1992;8:166-172

[40] Lazarides AL Alentorn-Geli E Choi JHJ, et al. Rotator cuff tears in young patients: A different disease than rotator cuff tears in elderly patients. Journal of Shoulder and Elbow Surgery. 2015;24(11):1834-1843

[41] Clement, et al. Sports medicine arthroscopy rehabilitation. Therapy & Technology. 2012;4:48

[42] Tashijan RZ. Epidemiology, natural history and indications for treatment of rotator cuff tears. Clinics in Sports Medicine. 2012;31(4):589-604

[43] Abdulwahab T, Betancourt J, Hassan F. Initial treatment of complete rotator cuff tear and transition to surgical treatment: Systematic review of the evidence. Muscles, Ligaments and Tendons Journal. 2016;6(1):35-47

[44] Heerspink FOL, Raay JJV, Koorevaar RC, Eerden PJV, Westerbeek RE, van't Riet E, et al. Comparing surgical repair with conservative treatment for degenerative rotator cuff tears: A randomized controlled trial. Journal of Shoulder and Elbow Surgery. 2015;24:1274-1281

[45] Shibany Hibany N, Zehetgruber H, Kainberger F, et al. Rotator cuff tears in asymptoatic individuals: A clinical and ultrasonographic screeening study. European Journal of Radiology. 2004;51(3):263-268

[46] Schibany N, Zehetgruber H, Kainberger F, Wurnig C, Ba-Ssalamah A, Herneth A, et al. Rotator cuff tears in asymptomatic individuals: A clinical and ultrasonographic screening study. European Journal of Radiology. 2004;**51**:263-268

[47] Kukkonen J, Joukainen A, Lehtinen J, Mattila K.T, Tuominen EKJ, Kauko T, Aarimaa V. Treatment of non-traumatic rotator cuff tears A randomised controlled trials with one year clinical results. The Bone and Joint Journal. 2014;**96**(1):75-81

[48] Ainsworth R, Lewis J, Conboy V. A prospective randomised placebo controlled clinical trial of a rehabilitation programme for patients with a diagnosis of massive rotator cuff tears of the shoulder. Journal of the British Elbow and Shoulder Society. 2009;**1**:55-60

[49] Levy O, Mllett H, Roberts S, Copeland S. The role of anterior deltoid reeducation in patients with massive irreparable degenerative rotator cuff tears. Journal of Shoulder and Elbow Surgery. 2008;**17**:863-870

[50] Koubaa S, Ben Salah FZ, Lebib S, et al. Conservative management of full thickness rotator cuff tears: A prospective study of 24 patients. Annales de Réadaptation et de Médecine Physique. 2006;**6**(2):24-27

[51] Ainsworth R. Physiotherapy rehabilitation in patients with massive, irreparable rotator cuff tears. Musculoskeletal Care. 2006;**4**(3):140-151

[52] Gagey O, Hue E. Mechanics of the deltoid muscle. A new approach. Clinical Orthopaedics. 2000;**375**:250-257

[53] Moseley GL. Combined physiotherapy and education is effective for chronic low back pain. A randomised controlled trial. Australian Journal of Physiotherapy. 2002;**48**:297-302

[54] Moseley GL. Joining forces – combining cognition-targeted motor control training with group or individual pain physiology education: A successful treatment for chronic low back pain. The Journal of Manual and Manipulative Therapy. 2003;**11**:88-89

[55] Kuhn JE, Dunn WR, Sanders R, et al. Effectiveness of physical therapy in treating atraumatic full-thickness rotator cuff tears: A multicenter prospective cohort study. Journal of Shoulder and Elbow Surgery. 2013;**22**:1371-1379

[56] Edwards P, Ebert J, Joss B, Bhabra G, Ackland T, Wang A. Exercise rehabilitation in the non-operative management of rotator cuff tears: A review of the literature. The International Journal of Sports Physical Therapy. 2016;**11**(2):279-294

[57] Andres BM, Murrell GA. Treatment of tendinopathy: What works, what does not, and what is on the horizon. Clinical Orthopaedics and Related Research. 2008;**466**:1539-1554

[58] Boudreault J, Desmeules F, Roy J, Dionne C, Fremont P, Macdermid J. The efficacy of oral non-steroidal anti-inflammatory drugs for rotator cuff tendinopathy: A systematic review and meta-analysis. Journal of Rehabilitation Medicine. 2014;**46**(4):294-306

[59] Nakamura H, Gotoh M, Kanazawa T, Ohta K, Nakamura K, Honda H, et al. Effects of corticosteroids and hyaluronic acid on torn rotator cuff tendons in vitro and in rats. Journal of Orthopaedic Research. 2015;**33**(10):1523-1530

[60] Shibata Y, Midorikawa K, Emoto G, Naito M. Clinical evaluation of sodium hyaluronate for the treatment of patients with rotator cuff tears. Journal of Shoulder and Elbow Surgery. 2001;**19**(1):116-120

[61] Blaine T, Moskowitz R, Udell J, et al. Treatment of persistent shoulder pain with sodium hyaluronate: A randomized, controlled trial. The Journal of Bone and Joint Surgery. American Volume. 2008;**90**(5):970-979

[62] Costantino C, Ovirri S. Rehabilitative and infiltrative treatment with hyaluronic acid in elderly patients with rotator cuff tears. Acta Biomed. 2009;**80**(3):225-229

[63] Gialanella B, Bertolinelli B. Corticosteroids injection in rotator cuff tears in elderly patient: Pain outcome prediction. Geriatrics and Gerontology International Journal. 2013;**13**(4):993-1001

[64] Caplan Al. Mesenchymal stem cells. Journal of Orthopaedic Research. 1991;**9**:641-650

[65] Amable P, Carias R, Teixeira M, da Cruz Pacheco Í, Corrêa do Amaral R, Granjeiro J, et al. Platelet-rich plasma preparation for regenerative medicine: Optimization and quantification of cytokines and growth factors. Stem Cell Research & Therapy. 2013;**4**(3):67

[66] Mehta S, Watson JT. Platelet-rich concentrate: Basic science and clinical applications. Journal of Orthopaedic Trauma. 2008;**22**:432-438

[67] Bennett NT, Schultz GS. Growth factors and wound healing: Biochemical properties of growth factors and their receptors. American Journal of Surgery. 1993;**165**:728-737

[68] Zhang J, Wang J. Platelet-rich releasate promotes differentiation of tendon stem cells in tendon cells. The American Journal of Sports Medicine. 2010;**38**:2477-2486

[69] Takase F, Inui A, Mifune Y, Sakata R, Muto T, Harada Y, Ueda Y, Kokubu T, Kurosaka M. Effect of platelet-rich plasma on degeneration change of rotator cuff muscles: In vitro and in vivo evaluations. Journal of Orthopaedic Research. 2017

[70] Boswell SG, Cole BJ, Sundman EA, Karas V, Fortier LA. Platelet-rich plasma: A milieu of bioactive factors. Arthroscopy. 2012;**28**:429-439

[71] Hall MP, Band PA, Meislin RJ, Jazrawi LM, Cardone DA. Platelet-rich plasma: Current concepts and application in sports medicine. The Journal of the American Academy of Orthopaedic Surgeons. 2009;**17**:602-608

[72] Crisan M, Yap S, Casteila L, et al. A perivascular origin for mesenchymal stem cells in multiple human organs. Cell Stem Cell. 2008;**3**:301-313

[73] Cesselli D, Beltrami AP, Rigo S, et al. Multipotent progenitor cells are present in human peripheral blood. Circulation Research. 2009;**104**:1225-1234

[74] Murphy MB, Moncivais K, Caplan AL. Mesenchymal stem cells: Environmentally responsive therapeutics for regenerative medicine. Experimental & Molecular Medicine. 2013;**45**:e54

[75] Jo C, Kim J, Yoon K, Shin S. Platelet-rich plasma stimulates cell proliferation and enhances matrix gene expression and synthesis in tenocytes from human rotator cuff tendons with degenerative tears. The American Journal of Sports Medicine. 2012;**40**(5):1035-1045

[76] Beck J, Evans D, Tonino PM, Yong S, Callaci JJ. The biomechanical and histologic effects of platelet-rich plasma on rat rotator cuff repairs. The American Journal of Sports Medicine. 2012;**40**:2037-2044

[77] Gumina S, Campagna V, Ferrazza G, Giannicola G, Fratalocchi F, Milani A, Postacchini F. Use of platelet-leukocyte membrane in arthroscopic repair of large rotator cuff tears. The Journal of Bone and Joint Surgery-American Volume. 2012;94(15):1345-1352

[78] Caplan Al. All MSCs are pericytes? Cell Stem Cell. 2008;**3**:229-230

[79] Heringou P, Flouzat Lachaniette CH, Delambre J, et al. Biologic augmentation of rotator cuff repair with mesenchymal stem cells during arthroscopy improves healing and prevents further tears: A case-controlled study. International Orthopaedics. 2014;**38**:1811-1818

[80] Sambandam SN, Khanna V, Gul A, Mornasamy V. Rotator cuff tears: An evidence based approach. World Journal of Orthopedics. 2015;**6**(11):902-918. DOI: 10.5312/wjo.v6.i11.902

[81] Tanaka M, Itoi E, Sato K, Hamada J, Hitachi S, Tojo Y, Tabata S. Factors related to successful outcome of conservative treatment for rotator cuff tears. Upsala Journal of Medical Sciences. 2010;**115**:193-200

[82] Hsu J, Keener J. Natural history of rotator cuff disease and implications on management. Operative Techniques in Orthopaedics. 2015;**25**:1-9. DOI: 10.1053/j.oto.2014.11.006

[83] Reilly P, Macleod I, Macfarlane R, Windley J, Emery RJ. Dead men and radiologists don't lie: A review of cadaveric and radiological studies of rotator cuff tear prevalence. Annals of the Royal College of Surgeons of England. 2006;**88**:116-121

[84] Sher JS, Uribe JW, Posada A. Abnormal findings on magnetic resonance images of asymptomatic shoulders. The Journal of Bone and Joint Surgery. American Volume. 1995;**77**:10-15

[85] Moosmayer S, Smith HJ, Tariq R, Larmo A. Prevalence and characteristics of asymptomatic tears of the rotator cuff: An ultrasonographic and clinical study. The Journal of Bone and Joint Surgery. British Volume. 2009;**91**(2):196-200

[86] Baydar M, Akalin E, El O, Gulbahar S, Bircan C, Akgul O, Manisali M, Torun Orhan B, Kizil R. The efficacy of conservative treatment in patients with full-thickness rotator cuff tears. Rheumatology International. 2008;29(6):623-628

[87] Dunn WR, Schackman BR, Walsh C, et al. Variation in orthopaedic surgeons' perceptions about the indications for rotator cuff surgery. The Journal of Bone and Joint Surgery. American Volume. 2005;**87**(9):1978-1984

[88] Kweon C, Gagnier J, Robbins C, Bedi A, Carpenter J, Miller B. Surgical versus nonsurgical management of rotator cuff tears: Predictors of treatment allocation. The American Journal of Sports Medicine. 2015;**43**(10):2368-2372

[89] Björnsson H, Norlin R, Johansson K, Adolfsson L. The influence of age, delay of repair, and tendon involvement in acute rotator cuff tears. Acta Orthopaedica. 2011;**82**(2):187-192

[90] Merolla G, Paladini P, Saporito M, Porcellini G. Conservative management of rotator cuff tears: Literature review and proposal for a prognostic. Prediction Score. Muscles Ligaments Tendons Journal. 2011;**1**(1):12-19

[91] Schmidt C, Morrey B. Management of full-thickness rotator cuff tears: Appropriate use criteria. Journal of Shoulder and Elbow Surgery. 2017;**24**(12):1860-1867

[92] Paxton ES, Teefey SA, Dahiya N, Keener JD, Yamaguchi K, Galatz LM. Clinical and radiographic outcomes of failed repairs of large or massive rotator cuff tears: Minimum ten-year follow-up. The Journal of Bone and Joint Surgery. American Volume. 2013 Apr 3;**95**(7):627-632

[93] Walch G, Edwards TB, Boulahia A, Nové-Josserand L, Neyton L, Szabo I. Arthroscopic tenotomy of the long head of the biceps in the treatment of rotator cuff tears: Clinical and radiographic results of 307 cases. Journal of Shoulder and Elbow Surgery. 2005 May–Jun;**14**(3):238-246

[94] Park JG, Cho NS, Song JH, Baek JH, Jeong HY, Rhee YG. Rotator cuff repair in patients over 75 years of age: Clinical outcome and repair integrity. Clinics in Orthopedic Surgery. 2016 Dec;**8**(4):420-427

[95] Wirth MA, Basamania C, Rockwood CA. Nonoperative management of full-thickness tears of the rotator cuff. The Orthopedic Clinics of North America. 1997;**28**(1):59-67

[96] Boorman RS, More KD, Hollinshead RM, Wiley JP, Brett K, Mohtadi NG, Nelson AA, Lo IK, Bryant D. The rotator cuff quality-of-life index predicts the outcome of nonoperative treatment of patients with a chronic rotator cuff tear. The Journal of Bone and Joint Surgery. American Volume. 2014;**96**(22):1883-1888

6

Current Outcomes Following Reverse Total Shoulder Arthroplasty

Sydney C. Cryder, Samuel E. Perry and
Elizabeth A. Beverly

Abstract

Reverse Total Shoulder Arthroplasty (RTSA) is a popular treatment for patients with rotator cuff damage, glenohumeral arthritis, complex fractures, and previously failed total shoulder arthroplasty given its ability to alleviate pain and increase range of motion and function. Although RTSA significantly improves functionality, pain, and satisfaction, patients need to be given realistic expectations for when to expect improvements, peak performance, and plateaus as well as potential risks for negative outcomes. As with any surgical procedure, patients are at risk for intraoperative, perioperative, short-term, and long-term complications. Thus, the purpose of this review is to discuss the short-term and long-term complications, metrics, and length of follow-up for patients who have undergone RTSA. In addition, we provide recommendations for a cut-off point between short-term and long-term outcomes for RTSA.

Keywords: reverse total shoulder arthroplasty, joint prosthesis, shoulder joint surgery, rotator cuff surgery, short-term outcomes, long-term outcomes

1. Introduction

In 1985, Dr. Paul Grammont introduced a new system for reverse total shoulder prosthesis that revolutionized the field by focusing on four key features: (1) the prosthesis must be inherently stable; (2) the lever arm of the deltoid must be effective from the initiation of the movement; (3) the glenosphere must be large and the humeral cup small to create a semi-constrained articulation; (4) the center of rotation must be fixed, medialized and distalized with respect to the glenoid surface [1, 2]. To this day, Grammont's core features are still the mainstay. Of course, modern prosthetics have been modified since 1985 to avoid scapular notching and impingement between the greater tuberosity and the coracoacromial arch and to maximize compressive forces while minimizing shear forces [2, 3].

These advancements contributed directly to the increased utilization of Reverse Total Shoulder Arthroplasty (RTSA) [4]. In fact, in the last ten years, the number of RTSAs nearly tripled in the United States [5]. Reverse Total Shoulder Arthroplasty (RTSA) is a popular treatment for patients with rotator cuff damage, glenohumeral arthritis, complex fractures, and previously failed total shoulder arthroplasty given its ability to alleviate pain and increase range of motion and function. Although RTSA significantly improves functionality, pain, and satisfaction, patients need to be given realistic expectations for when to expect improvements, peak performance, and plateaus as well as potential risks for negative outcomes. As with any surgical procedure, patients are at risk for intraoperative, perioperative, short-term, and long-term complications. Thus, the purpose of this review is to discuss the short-term and long-term complications, metrics, and length of follow-up for patients who have undergone RTSA. In addition, we provide recommendations for a cut-off point between short-term and long-term outcomes for RTSA.

Ease range of motion and function in patients with glenohumeral joint disease, displaced proximal humeral fractures, rotator cuff tear arthropathy, severe irreparable rotator cuff tears, rheumatoid arthritis, and failed shoulder arthroplasty [1–3, 6–8].

2. Surgical approach

The surgical technique for RTSA can be accomplished via two approaches: deltopectorally or superolaterally [3, 9]. The deltopectoral approach is the most common and requires an experienced surgeon [10]. This surgical technique begins with an incision overlying the deltopectoral interval, preserving the cephalic vein, then tenotomizing the biceps tendon and the subscapularis if still intact [3, 11, 12]. Next, the joint capsule is circumferentially released and humeral head exposed to perform a humeral head osteotomy. The humeral head is then reamed and broached. Subsequently, the glenoid is exposed, the labrum excised, and the glenoid prepared. The guidewire for the glenoid reamer is placed inferiorly so that the glenoid baseplate will be flush with the inferior border of the native glenoid rim. This will help decrease the risk of scapular notching. By adding an inferior tilt to the position of the baseplate, the risk of scapular notching can be decreased, which in turn, improves compressive forces and helps avoid shear forces on the glenoid component. The baseplate is impacted in place, and secured with screws to securely fix the baseplate to the patient's native glenoid. The selected glenosphere is then secured to the baseplate with a Morse Taper fixation mechanism. The selection of the appropriately sized glenosphere is multifactorial. It is based on the patient's size (i.e., 42 mm for larger patients, 39 mm for average size patients, 36 mm for smaller patients) and individual patient pathologies. Glenosphere components are available in central, lateral offset, and inferior offset designs.

Next, the humeral stem is prepared by sounding the inner diameter of the humeral shaft and broaching it to the appropriate size. The final implant is tested with the spacer trials in order to gain proper stability and range of motion. Then the real implants are seated and the shoulder is reduced. Lastly, the subscapularis is reattached and the biceps are tenodesed with heavy nonabsorbable sutures that are placed through drill holes in the humeral metaphysis prior to seating of the final implant. However, recent research acknowledges the controversy surrounding the reattachment of the subscapularis due to the potential for increasing the likelihood of dislocation [13]. The deltopectoral-interval is re-approximated and the incision closed. The patient is placed in a shoulder abduction sling for a period of immobilization lasting two to 6 weeks with a home physical therapy program [14]. As with all orthopedic procedures, the rehabilitation protocol is patient specific and additional rehabilitation may be deemed necessary if the patient needs to strengthen external rotation [14].

3. Outcome timeline

What constitutes a short-term versus a long-term outcome? One of the objectives of this review is to address the lack of clarity in the literature regarding the timeline of short-term and long-term outcomes [15]. Bacle and colleagues [15] identified that the majority of mechanical loosening reports occurred outside of the first 2 years following a reverse total shoulder arthroplasty. In contrast, dislocation, infection, and poor seating of the glenoid component were reported within the first 2 years postoperatively; a ratio of 3 to 1 for complications reported before and after the two-year mark [15]. Furthermore, Bacle and colleagues [15] defined medium-term follow-up as a mean of 39 months and long-term follow-up as a mean of 150 months. Similarly, Otto and colleagues [16] argued that a follow-up of period of 24 months was a relatively short time frame to adequately capture long-term complications. Thus, 2 years may be a respectable partition between short-term and long-term outcomes.

4. Outcome quantification

The language of RTSA outcomes is a complex task given the wide range of outcomes metrics. The most common scoring methods include the following: Range of Motion (ROM), Constant-Murley Score (CMS), American Surgeons of Elbow and Shoulder score (ASES), Visual Analogue Score (VAS), and the Simple Shoulder Test (SST). Other methods include but are not limited to the UCLA Shoulder Score and the Shoulder Pain and Disability Index (SPADI) [17–19]. The CMS, first published in 1987, is comprised of four sections: two of which are self-reported by the patient—pain and activities of daily living, the remaining two are reported by the physician—range of motion and strength [20]. Concerns were raised regarding the score's ability to account for age and gender; thus, the modified version adjusts for both [17]. The ASES was created with the goal of developing a universal outcome measure; it too contains patient-reported and physician-reported parts. In addition, the ASES has demonstrated appropriate validity and reliability in assessing operative and non-operative interventions for shoulder pathology [17]. However, it's appraisal of functionality may be somewhat limited among the older adult population; for example, the questions about "do usual sport" and "throw ball overhand" may not be relevant [19]. Patient-reported pain is an outcome that necessitates acknowledgement, which may be quantified by utilizing the VAS [21]. The VAS uses a line measuring 100 mm with pain extremes indicated on either end; no pain and worst pain [21]. The patient marks along the continuum where he/she believes their pain is best described; the score is then represented by a distance in millimeters [22]. Finally, the SST, is used to evaluate patient-reported functionality associated with various shoulder pathology, including rotator cuff arthropathy, osteoarthritis, rheumatoid arthritis, and adhesive capsulitis [17, 18]. This questionnaire consists of 12 questions that ask the patient whether he/she may perform the given activity [18].

5. Short-term outcomes

Table 1 reviews the outcome measures and length of follow-up from numerous surgical studies. Based on these findings, short-term outcomes for RTSA occur postoperatively within the first 24 months. It also addresses the variation in components and metrics used in each study.

RTSA significantly improves functionality, pain, and satisfaction; but when are patients expected to experience peak performance with a new prosthesis? Is there a point in time when a patient should expect a plateau in their improvements over time? In 2015, Simovitch and colleagues [23] demonstrated that at the 6-month follow-up, less than 5% of patients reported decreases in SST, UCLA Shoulder Score, CMS, ASES, SPADI. More importantly, "full improvement" was achieved in the 12–24 month range [23]. Thus, they concluded that the majority of improvement occurred within the first 6 months, as evidenced by the scores for each of the five measures [23]. These findings stress the importance of patient selection, expectations for RTSA, expertise in intraoperative optimization, and strict postoperative physical therapy management. The concept of rapid improvement during the first 6 months with plateau at 12 months was also reported by Muller and colleagues in 2017 [24], in which flexion, abduction, and external rotation in 90 degrees of abduction demonstrated profound increases by 42°, 38° and 33° respectively at 6 months. Additional follow-ups at 12, 24, and 60 months displayed minimal additional improvement [24]. Supplementary evidence of RTSA success was seen by Yoon and colleagues [25] in 2017 with forward flexion increase of 64°, external rotation increase of 13° and pain reduction of (−3) at 12 months postoperatively.

Two factors that have been shown to increase CMS and ROM testing during the short-term period are deltoid volume [25] and glenosphere size [24] respectively. Preoperative deltoid muscle volume was an independent prognostic factor for functional outcomes with CMS (p = 0.011), underscoring the importance of patient selection and discussing the potential for negative outcomes such as atrophied deltoid muscle [25]. Likewise, Muller and colleagues [24] conducted a retrospective analysis in 2017, to demonstrate that patients that had received a 44 mm glenosphere had greater external rotation in adduction and abduction strength over the 36 mm glenosphere. Moreover, they found no significant differences in functional scores or complication rates [24].

Study	Sample size	Age	Follow up	Complications	Component variability	Risk factors	Scoring Mechanism
Alentorn-Geli et al (2017)	38	77–83 years	3–60 months	Infection Glenoid loosening Revisions Component Dislocation	Comprehensive reverse shoulder system (Biomet) Encore reverse (DJO Global) Delta reverse shoulder System (DePuy)	Tobacco use Diabetes Mellitus Hypertension Increased age	FF ER
Anakwenze et al (2016)	1147	45–84 years	3–36 months	Aseptic revision Mortality Surgical site infection Readmission	-	Increased BMI Diabetes Mellitus Increased age	-
Bacle et al (2017)	186	23–86 years (72.7 mean)	24–150 months	Dislocation Scapular Notching Infection Nerve Palsy Glenoid Loosening Humeral Loosening Glenoid fracture Revisions	164 Delta III (DePuy) 27 Aequalis (Tournier)	Increased age	CMS ROM
Ek et al. (2013)	41	46–64 years	60–171 months	Infection Nerve Palsy Fracture Dislocation Component Wear Glenoid loosening	Glenoid component 36mm, 40mm, or 42 mm Delta III (DePuy) (lateralized humeral polyethylene cup) Anatomical Shoulder System (Zimmer) (6mm medialized humeral cup)	Previous surgery on same shoulder	CMS Validated electronic dynamometer
Feeley et al (2014)	54	53–81 years	30 months	Scapular notching	Zimmer Reverse Trabecular Metal System 36mm glenosphere 3mm lateralized	-	VAS ASES score ROM

Study	Sample size	Age	Follow up	Complications	Component variability	Risk factors	Scoring Mechanism
Friedman et al (2017)	591	50–93 years	24 month minimum (37 month mean)	Component instability Scapular notching	Equinoxe rTSA (Exactech)	-	SST ASES score UCLA score CMS SPADI
Jonusas et al (2017)	27	55–85 years	45 months	Heterotopic ossification Tubercule malposition	Arrow shoulder system with less medialized CoR	-	SST CMS
Mollon et al (2016)	476	53–90 years	22–93 months	Scapular notching Dislocation Infection Component Loosening Humeral fracture Scapular fracture	Equinoxe rTSA (Exactech) 36 mm, 40mm, or 42mm glenosphere lateralized 2.3mm	Increased age Increased BMI	ROM ASES score CMS SST
Muller et al (2017)	68	68–79 years	6–60 months	Glenoid migration Component loosening	SMR reverse shoulder system (Lima Switzerland SA) 36mm or 40mm glenosphere	Increased age	CMS SPADI
Otto et al. (2017)	67	21–54 years	24–144 months	Scapular notching Humeral lucency Glenoid screw lucency Fracture (humeral, scapular) Humeral dissociation Infection Instability Revision	Reverse shoulder system (DJO Surgical)	Prior shoulder surgery	SST ASES score
Randelli et al (2015)	226	64–72 years	3.8 years	Revision Infection Fracture	Delta III	-	Constant Score ASES score

Study	Sample size	Age	Follow up	Complications	Component variability	Risk factors	Scoring Mechanism
Simovitch et al (2015)	912	60–78 years	2 weeks–139 months	-	Equinoxe rTSA system (Exactech)	-	SPADI ASES score UCLA score Constant score
Statz et al (2016)	41	53–83 years	2–7.3 years	Scapular notching Revision Nerve palsy Heterotopic ossification	Encore reverse shoulder Prosthesis (DJO Surgical) Delta III, Delta Xtend (DePuy) Comprehensive prosthesis (Biomet) Aequalis Reversed Shoulder (Tournier)	Increased BMI Previous shoulder surgery Tobacco use Diabetes mellitus	ROM ASES score
Wierks et al (2007)	20	45–88 years	3–21 months	Fracture Poor screw fixation Nerve palsy Infection/ Abscess Dislocation Revision Heterotopic ossification Scapular notching	DePuy reverse shoulder prosthesis Tournier reverse shoulder prosthesis	-	-
Williams et al (2017)	17	45–91 years	10–67.7 months	Dislocation Component migration	Biomet reverse adapter (Bio-Modular to Comprehensive conversion)	-	VAS ASES score
Yoon et al (2017)	35	66–84 years	12–35 months	Scapular notching A/C joint separation Acromial fracture	Aequalis reverse arthroplasty system (Tournier)	Increase BMI Diabetes mellitus Hypertension Decreased BMD	VAS ASES score Constant score SST

ASES = American shoulder and elbow surgeons; SPADI = shoulder pain and disability index; ROM = range of motion; UCLA = University of California Los Angeles score; SST = simple shoulder test; VAS = visual analogue score; FF = forward flexion; ER = external rotation; BMD = bone mineral density.

Table 1. Comparison of outcome measures and length of follow-up for patients undergoing reverse total shoulder arthroplasty.

Complications are a critical component of RTSA. Patients need to be counseled on intraoperative, perioperative, and notably, short-term complications. The most common intraoperative complications are glenoid or humeral fractures along with poor screw fixation [12]. The consequence of poor screw fixation is its lasting impact and conversion to long-term complications such as glenoid screw lucency. Zhou and colleagues [13] discussed the prevention techniques, such as hand reaming the humerus and preserving glenoid bone stock by avoiding reaming beyond subchondral bone margin. Postoperative short-term complications dominate the outcomes of RTSA and range from scapular notching, infection, dislocation, revision, nerve palsy, or even heterotopic ossification.

Scapular notching is by far the most common complication during the first 24 months postoperative. Scapular notching has an incidence of 38%, 57%, 55% and 73% in four recent studies respectively [12, 15, 24, 25]. These findings oblige additional research to review instrumentation and confirm incidence levels on scapular notching in RTSA. In 2014, Feeley and colleagues [12] found that decreasing the neck-shaft angle or a higher inclination angle and 3 mm lateral offset of the glenosphere prosthesis decreased the rate of scapular notching by 16%. Furthermore, Zhou and colleagues [13] assert that continued complication management, by adding inferior placement of the glenosphere, is "the most important factor in the avoidance of inferior impingement." The next step is to investigate whether scapular notching will evolve, both de novo and from early to late stage scapular notching during short-term follow-up. An important question to consider is will the patient be free from scapular notching for the remainder of the prosthesis? [12] Feeley and colleagues [12] observed that of all the patients who did not experience scapular notching during the first 12 months (84% of patients), showed no new evidence of scapular notching during follow-ups up to 30 months. Conversely, Bacle and colleagues [15] found that after early scapular notching diagnoses were made, there was a 39% increase in the rate of notching beyond the 2-year follow-up period. Thus, superfluous research is essential to answer this question.

Another common short term complication deals with postoperative stability resulting in shoulder dislocations. Wierks [12] and colleagues as well as Bacle [15] and colleagues found 10% and 22% of dislocations occurred during the short term period. Of note, Bacle and colleagues [15] published that of the 15 dislocations documented in the sample size of 67, no cases were reported after the 2 year follow-up period. Zhou and colleagues [26] reviewed the most common and serious complications associated with RTSA and concluded that instability was a result of "lack of soft tissue tension, mechanical impingement, mismatch of the glenosphere and humeral socket size and improper version of the prosthesis". Therefore, to obtain the best outcome for patients, extensive knowledge of the prosthesis is imperative, along with understanding how to achieve soft tissue tension using vertical offset of your acromion—greater tuberosity distance and lateral offset of the tuberosity-glenoid distance [26]. Conversely, controversy exists within the RTSA literature regarding the decision to repair the subscapularis. Friedman and colleagues showed that subscapularis repair proclaimed no statistical significance over no repair [27]. In the study, 340 patients with RTSA plus repair had 0% dislocation rate, versus 251 patients with RTSA without repair showing a 1.2% dislocation rate; stating the claim that RTSA plus subscapularis repair is not indicated due to the absence of increase in overall complication rates [27].

Lastly, infections can have serious ramifications on patient satisfaction as well as the overall outcomes of the RTSA, resulting in one or two-stage revisions. A study conducted by Wierks and colleagues [12] in 2009, had a 5% infection rate and a study by Bacle and colleagues [15] in 2017, had an infection rate of 12%. It is important to emphasize that Bacle and colleagues [15] documented 8 infections within the first 24 months as compared to only 2 cases in the 12 year follow-up period. In the same study, with regards to revision cases in the short-term period, 6 out of the 8 revision surgeries were caused by infections [15]. Thus, postoperative infections that occur in the first two years are the most common reason for revision surgery. In the review conducted by Zhou and colleagues [26] in 2015, they compared primary cases and revision cases, to find that revision cases were statistically higher than primary cases with regards to infections rates, 5.9% vs. 2.9% respectively. *Propionibacterium acnes* and *Staphylococcus epidermidis* were the most commonly cultured organisms. Recommendations to decrease infections include continuation of preoperative antibiotics within one hour of incision and use of antibiotic-impregnated cement for surgeries that employ cement the humeral component [26].

6. Long-term outcomes

The patient's age at the time of the arthroplasty plays a critical role in the survival of the prosthesis; younger patients (i.e., < 55 years of age) are more likely to be active in the workforce, while older patients are less likely to participate in physically strenuous activities and be retired [16]. In younger patients, prosthesis survival can exceed 10 years. For example, Bacle and colleagues [15] observed a 93% implant survival rate at 10 years; whereas Ek and colleagues [28] observed an implant survival rate of 88% at 5 years and 76% at 10 years postoperatively, regardless of any complications that may have arisen.

The RTSA has been shown to improve pain, strength, range of motion in abduction, external rotation, and forward flexion; in addition to showing improvement in metrics, such as ASES, SST, CMS, SPADI, and UCLA Should and UCLA Shoulder Score [16, 23, 24, 29]. Outcomes beyond the 24-month mark may be impacted by multiple variables, some of which include, prosthesis sizes, involvement of fracture, primary versus revision RTSA, and the lifestyle or activity level of the patient. In regards to repair of proximal humeral fractures, RTSA was found to provide superior results to a hemiarthroplasty for at least 5 years, respectively [30]. Muller and colleagues [24] investigated the size of the glenosphere, 36 mm and 44 mm, on functional outcomes following RTSA and found that both groups exhibited the most substantial progress in the first 6–24 months, followed by a plateau. Patients' progress was monitored by measuring flexion, abduction, external rotation at 0° and 90° of abduction, internal rotation at 90° of abduction, CMS, SPADI, and strength (kg) in abduction. Interestingly, Anakwenze and colleagues [31] found that a higher body mass index (BMI) put a patient at risk for deep surgical site infection (SSI) up to 3 years following RTSA. Their study looked at the effects of increased BMI on postoperative outcomes following a RTSA and total shoulder arthroplasty (TSA). Every 5 kg/m [2] increase in BMI was associated with higher risk of 3-year deep SSI [31]. In addition to BMI, tobacco use influences the success of the prosthesis up to 12 years after an RTSA [32]. Hatta and colleagues [32] found that current smokers had an increased risk for infection, component loosening, and fractures compared to non-smokers. Specifically, they found that the percentage of patients with periprosthetic fractures jumped 20% at the 9 year mark after RTSA [32].

Although, as previously stated, this study implies 24 months as the short-term interval for outcomes following an RTSA, short-term complications have the potential to extend into the long-term if not addressed or managed appropriately—eventually affecting the longevity of the prosthesis. More commonly, long-term complications include glenoid and/or humeral component loosening, polyethylene component wear, and scapular notching. Less common long-term complications include deep SSI, dislocation, readmission, and fracture; which primarily occur within the first 2 years postoperatively. As mentioned above, glenoid or humeral loosening is the most common complication observed 2 years after RTSA, particularly with an increased risk following a previously failed shoulder arthroplasty and excess mechanical load related to increased BMI [15, 33]. Further, the incidence of component loosening doubles between the second and fifth year follow-up as reported by Alentorn-Geli and colleagues [29]. Particlization of the polyethylene component may be of concern with RTSA in younger patients due to necessary durability and lifespan of the implant. Riley and colleagues [34] investigated the outcomes following RTSA using a metal-on-metal design and concluded that it is not an acceptable alternative to RTSA in young patients; they maintain that the polyethylene component is the more suitable option. Ek and colleagues [28] conducted a study evaluating RTSA in patients younger than 65 years of age using two groups: revision RTSA and primary RTSA. This study observed an increased incidence of scapular notching at less than 12 months follow-up and greater than 10 years follow-up; with 56% of patients experiencing some degree of scapular notching overall [28]. Conversely, Mollon and colleagues [34] reported that only 10% of patients experienced scapular notching; noting that risk factors for scapular notching included lower body weight, lower BMI, and RTSA on the non-dominant upper extremity. It is also worth mentioning the correlation between longer-term follow-up and increasing incidence of scapular notching [34]; which may be attributed to variation in size and placement of the glenosphere, and center of rotation of the prosthesis.

7. Conclusion

Throughout this literature review, several limitations were encountered that include the following: unspecified "normal" postoperative physical rehabilitation protocols, risk factors pertinent to specific complications, and lack of research investigating the long term outcomes for RTSA. Additional research is needed to examine the aforementioned limitations to enhance future outcomes following RTSA.

Scapular notching, dislocations, and infections lead the forefront of persistent complications for RTSA. As evidenced in this literature review, the vast majority of improvement plateaus around 6 to 24 months. Thus, patient optimization may be accomplished by implementing a short-term course of preoperative physical therapy focused on shoulder girdle strength. Further, numerous inconsistencies and contradictions were observed in the literature regarding the impact of BMI on RTSA outcomes. Research requires further confirmatory evidence before making any strong conclusions about limiting the use of RTSA in patients with increased BMI. On the other hand, tobacco use negatively impacts the outcomes following RTSA by nearly doubling the overall complication rate.

Author details

Sydney C. Cryder[1]*, Samuel E. Perry[2] and Elizabeth A. Beverly[3]

*Address all correspondence to: sc323908@ohio.edu

1 Department of Medicine, Ohio University, Heritage College of Osteopathic Medicine, Athens, United States

2 Department of Graduate Medical Education, Adena Health System, Chillicothe, United States

3 Department of Family Medicine, Ohio University, Heritage College of Osteopathic Medicine, Athens, United States

References

[1] Berliner JL, Regalado-Magdos A, Ma CB, Feeley BT. Biomechanics of reverse total shoulder arthroplasty. Journal Of Shoulder And Elbow Surgery/American Shoulder And Elbow Surgeons...[et al.]. Jan 2015;**24**(1):150-160

[2] Nam D, Kepler CK, Neviaser AS, et al. Reverse total shoulder arthroplasty: Current concepts, results, and component wear analysis. The Journal Of Bone And Joint Surgery. American volume. Dec 2010;**92**(Suppl 2):23-35

[3] Schairer WW, Nwachukwu BU, Lyman S, Craig EV, Gulotta LV. National utilization of reverse total shoulder arthroplasty in the United States. Journal Of Shoulder And Elbow Surgery/American Shoulder And Elbow Surgeon. Jan 2015;**24**(1):91-97

[4] Westermann RW, Pugely AJ, Martin CT, Gao Y, Wolf BR, Hettrich CM. Reverse shoulder Arthroplasty in the United States: A comparison of National Volume, patient demographics, complications, and surgical indications. The Iowa Orthopaedic Journal. 2015;**35**:1-7

[5] Wiater BP, Baker EA, Salisbury MR, et al. Elucidating trends in revision reverse total shoulder arthroplasty procedures: A retrieval study evaluating clinical, radiographic, and functional outcomes data. Journal Of Shoulder And Elbow Surgery/American Shoulder And Elbow Surgeon. Jul 2015;**24**(12):1915-1925

[6] Middernacht B, Van Tongel A, De Wilde LA. Critical review on prosthetic features available for reversed Total shoulder Arthroplasty. Biomed Research International. 2016;**2016**:3256931

[7] Jo SH, Kim JY, Cho NS, Rhee YG. Reverse Total shoulder Arthroplasty: Salvage procedure for failed prior Arthroplasty. Clinics In Orthopedic Surgery. Jun 2017;**9**(2):200-206

[8] Dilisio MF, Miller LR, Siegel EJ, Higgins LD. Conversion to Reverse Shoulder Arthroplasty: Humeral Stem Retention Versus Revision. Orthopedics. Sep 1 2015;**38**(9):e773-e779

[9] Gadea F, Bouju Y, Berhouet J, Bacle G, Favard L. Deltopectoral approach for shoulder arthroplasty: Anatomic basis. International Orthopaedics. Feb 2015;39(2):215-225

[10] Gerber BS, Brodsky IG, Lawless KA, et al. Implementation and evaluation of a low-literacy diabetes education computer multimedia application. Diabetes Care. Jul 2005; 28(7):1574-1580

[11] Wierks C, Skolasky RL, Ji JH, McFarland EG. Reverse total shoulder replacement: Intraoperative and early postoperative complications. Clinical Orthopaedics And Related Research. Jan 2009;467(1):225-234

[12] Zhou HS, Chung JS, Yi PH, Li X, Price MD. Management of complications after reverse shoulder arthroplasty. Current Reviews In Musculoskeletal Medicine. Mar 2015;8(1): 92-97

[13] Jarrett CD, Brown BT, Schmidt CC. Reverse shoulder arthroplasty. The Orthopedic Clinics of North America. Jul 2013;44(3):389-408 x

[14] Bacle G, Nove-Josserand L, Garaud P, Walch G. Long-Term Outcomes of Reverse Total Shoulder Arthroplasty: A Follow-up of a Previous Study. The Journal of Bone And Joint Surgery. American volume. Mar 15 2017;99(6):454-461

[15] Otto RJ, Virani NA, Levy JC, Nigro PT, Cuff DJ, Frankle MA. Scapular fractures after reverse shoulder arthroplasty: Evaluation of risk factors and the reliability of a proposed classification. Journal Of Shoulder And Elbow Surgery/American Shoulder And Elbow Surgeons. Nov 2013;22(11):1514-1521

[16] Wylie JD, Beckmann JT, Granger E, Tashjian RZ. Functional outcomes assessment in shoulder surgery. World Journal of Orthopedics. Nov 18 2014;5(5):623-633

[17] Roy JS, Macdermid JC, Goel D, Faber KJ, Athwal GS, Drosdowech DS. What is a successful outcome following reverse Total shoulder Arthroplasty? The Open Orthopaedics Journal. 2010;4:157-163

[18] Booker S, Alfahad N, Scott M, Gooding B, Wallace WA. Use of scoring systems for assessing and reporting the outcome results from shoulder surgery and arthroplasty. World Journal Of Orthopedics. Mar 18 2015;6(2):244-251

[19] Conboy VB, Morris RW, Kiss J, Carr AJ. An evaluation of the constant-Murley shoulder assessment. The Journal of Bone And Joint Surgery. British volume. Mar 1996;78(2): 229-232

[20] McCormack HM, Horne DJ, Sheather S. Clinical applications of visual analogue scales: A critical review. Psychological Medicine. Nov 1988;18(4):1007-1019

[21] MacDermid JC, Solomon P, Prkachin K. The Shoulder Pain and Disability Index demonstrates factor, construct and longitudinal validity. BMC Musculoskeletal Disorders. Feb 10 2006;7:12

[22] Simovitch R, Flurin PH, Marczuk Y, et al. Rate of improvement in clinical outcomes with anatomic and reverse Total shoulder Arthroplasty. Bulletin of the Hospital for Joint Disease. Dec 2015;73(Suppl 1):S111-S117

[23] Muller AM, Born M, Jung C, et al. Glenosphere size in reverse shoulder arthroplasty: Is larger better for external rotation and abduction strength? Journal Of Shoulder And Elbow Surgery/American Shoulder and Elbow Surgeons. Jul 24 2017

[24] Yoon JP, Seo A, Kim JJ, et al. Deltoid muscle volume affects clinical outcome of reverse total shoulder arthroplasty in patients with cuff tear arthropathy or irreparable cuff tears. PLoS One. 2017;**12**(3):e0174361

[25] Feeley BT, Zhang AL, Barry JJ, et al. Decreased scapular notching with lateralization and inferior baseplate placement in reverse shoulder arthroplasty with high humeral inclination. International Journal Of Shoulder Surgery. Jul 2014;**8**(3):65-71

[26] Friedman LG, Griesser MJ, Miniaci AA, Jones MH. Recurrent instability after revision anterior shoulder stabilization surgery. Arthroscopy. The Journal Of Arthroscopic & Related Surgery: Official Publication Of The Arthroscopy Association of North America and the International Arthroscopy Association. Mar 2014;**30**(3):372-381

[27] Ek ET, Neukom L, Catanzaro S, Gerber C. Reverse total shoulder arthroplasty for massive irreparable rotator cuff tears in patients younger than 65 years old: Results after five to fifteen years. Journal Of Shoulder And Elbow Surgery/American Shoulder And Elbow Surgeons. Sep 2013;**22**(9):1199-1208

[28] Alentorn-Geli E, Clark NJ, Assenmacher AT, et al. What Are the Complications, Survival, and Outcomes After Revision to Reverse Shoulder Arthroplasty in Patients Older Than 80 Years? Clinical Orthopaedics And Related Research. Jul 2017;**475**(11):2744-2751

[29] Boyle MJ, Youn SM, Frampton CM, Ball CM. Functional outcomes of reverse shoulder arthroplasty compared with hemiarthroplasty for acute proximal humeral fractures. Journal Of Shoulder And Elbow Surgery/American Shoulder And Elbow Surgeons. Jan 2013;**22**(1):32-37

[30] Eneanya ND, Goff SL, Martinez T, et al. Shared decision-making in end-stage renal disease: A protocol for a multi-center study of a communication intervention to improve end-of-life care for dialysis patients. BMC Palliative Care. 2015;**14**:30

[31] Hatta T, Werthel JD, Wagner ER, et al. Effect of smoking on complications following primary shoulder arthroplasty. Journal Of Shoulder And Elbow Surgery/American Shoulder And Elbow Surgeons. Jan 2017;**26**(1):1-6

[32] Statz JM, Schoch BS, Sanchez-Sotelo J, Sperling JW, Cofield RH. Shoulder arthroplasty for locked anterior shoulder dislocation: A role for the reversed design. International Orthopaedics. Jun 2017;**41**(6):1227-1234

[33] Riley C, Idoine J, Shishani Y, Gobezie R, Edwards B. Early Outcomes Following Metal-on-Metal Reverse Total Shoulder Arthroplasty in Patients Younger Than 50 Years. Orthopedics. Sep 01 2016;**39**(5):e957-e961

[34] Mollon B, Mahure SA, Roche CP, Zuckerman JD. Impact of scapular notching on clinical outcomes after reverse total shoulder arthroplasty: An analysis of 476 shoulders. Journal Of Shoulder And Elbow Surgery/American Shoulder And Elbow Surgeons. Jul 2017;**26**(7):1253-1261

7

Subscapularis Repair

Omkar P. Kulkarni and Satish B. Sonar

Abstract

Subscapularis is largest muscle of the rotator cuff. It is important component of shoulder joint for necessary of unimpaired shoulder movements. Since past decade subscapularis tears are recognized as source of pain and dysfunction of shoulder joint. New diagnostic techniques and arthroscopic repair surgeries help to treat subscapularis tears. This article provides an overview of types of tear, diagnostic methods and treatment options.

Keywords: rotator cuff, subscapularis tendon tear, subscapularis repair

1. Introduction

Rotator cuff consists of four muscles supraspinatus, infraspinatus, teres minor and subscapularis. Subscapularis is largest of the four and is attached to the Lesser Tubercle. It constitutes 50–60% of the rotator cuff. It is one of the main anterior stabilizers of the shoulder.

The subscapularis muscle is the primary internal rotator of the shoulder joint. It also gives strong anterior stability along with capsulolabral tissues to prevent anterior dislocation. Recent studies have shown how the subscapularis works together with the infraspinatus muscle to create smooth balancing force couple and provides concentric compression effect.

Subscapularis tears are not as common as tears of the supraspinatus tendon. Subscapularis tendon tears may be isolated or in conjunction with supraspinatus and infraspinatus tendon tears or biceps tear/ subluxation (**Figure 1**).

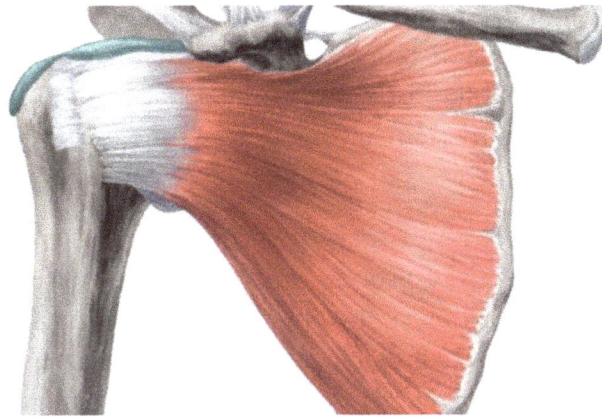

Figure 1. Subscapularis anatomy.

2. Overview

Subscapularis tendon tears have been firstly described by Smith [1] and Codman [2] Hauser reported in 1954 the first case of surgical repair of the subscapularis tendon [3].

Subscapularis tendon tears may be partial or full thickness. Chronic overload or acute trauma may cause tears. Traumatic tears are usually secondary to a forced external rotation or extension of the shoulder with the arm abducted. These tears are more prevalent in young patients as a consequence of a shoulder dislocation [4, 5]. In chronic tears due to repeated micro trauma degeneration, there is always an associated supraspinatus tear and biceps tendinosis or subluxation along with subscapularis tear. In tears of long duration, there can be severe retraction of the tendon underneath coracoids process. Sometimes it get tucked to superior capsule or glenohumeral ligaments forming a "Coma sign/tissue" as described by Burkhart [6].

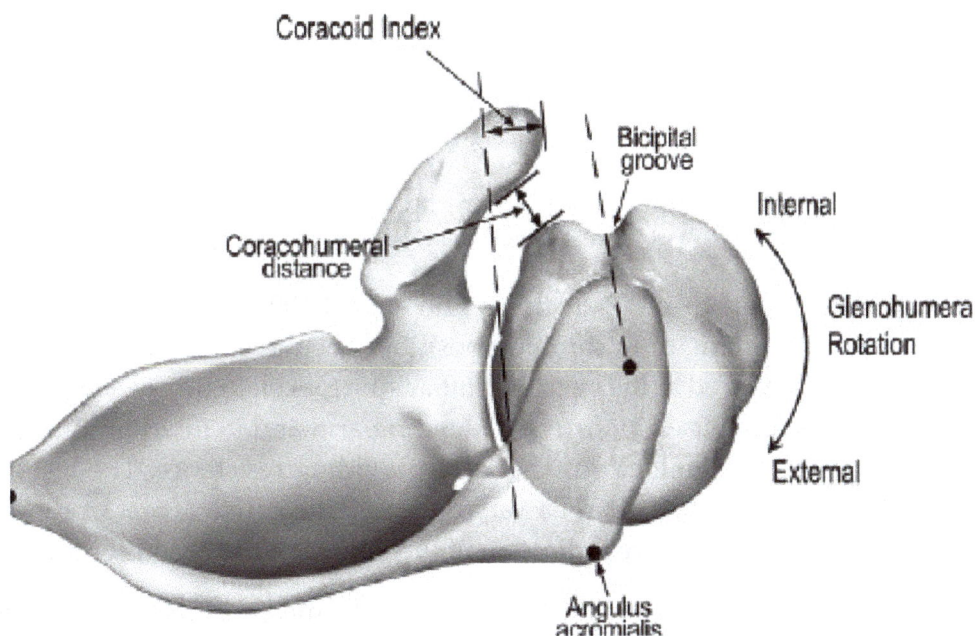

Figure 2. Coracoid impingement.

The main causes for subscapularis tear with or without other lesions is Sub coracoid impingement with reduced coracohumeral distance. Due to repeated friction in narrow canal beneath the coracoids process, attritional tear of subscapularis happens. When this distance, which normally ranges from 8.7 to 11 mm, is lower than 5 mm, the risk that the subscapularis tendon is torn is high [7, 8].

The coracoid impingement may be primary or acquired. Primary causes of sub coracoid impingement are lateralized coracoid process, calcifications or ossifications of the subscapularis tendon, subscapularis muscle hypertrophy, and ganglion cysts. Secondary causes are usually traumatic or degenerative like displaced humeral or scapular fractures, non-unions, posterior dislocation of the sternoclavicular joint, spur formation, etc., (**Figure 2**).

The subscapularis tendon is torn in 63% of patients in whom the biceps tendon is sub-luxated or dislocated as there is continuity between medial margin of pulley and the subscapularis tendon.

3. Symptoms

The shoulder pain related to a subscapularis tendon tear is more anterior compared to the typical pain observed in patients with rotator cuff tears. There is weakness in internal rotation and abduction like buttoning the shirt, adjusting the tie, tucking the shirt in the back etc. as these functions requires active internal rotation. Since in most of the cases anterior supraspinatus and biceps tendon is also involved, forward flexion, supination and abduction- external rotation can also be painful.

4. Clinical examination

On examination there will be increased passive external rotation, Loss of active internal rotation strength.

Lift-off, belly-press, Napoleon and bear-hug are specific tests to assess the subscapularis tendon.

The lift-off test: This test has 15–20% sensitivity and almost 100% specificity (Barth et al.) [9]. This test is carried out in sitting or in standing position. The patient's arm is kept in internal rotation with the hand is placed at the back at lumbar spine level. In this position patient tries to move the hand away from back by further extending arm and in internal rotation. Now if this movement is possible, examiner can check by providing resistance. The test is positive when the patient is unable to lift the hand away from back indicative of tear of subscapularis. The degree of weakness and pain are indicative of the degree of the lesion (**Figure 3**).

The belly-press test: It is one of the most commonly performed and accurate clinical test for subscapularis tear with sensitivity of 40% and specificity of 97.3%.It is also called as abdominal compression test, In this test patient attempts to press the hand against the belly with

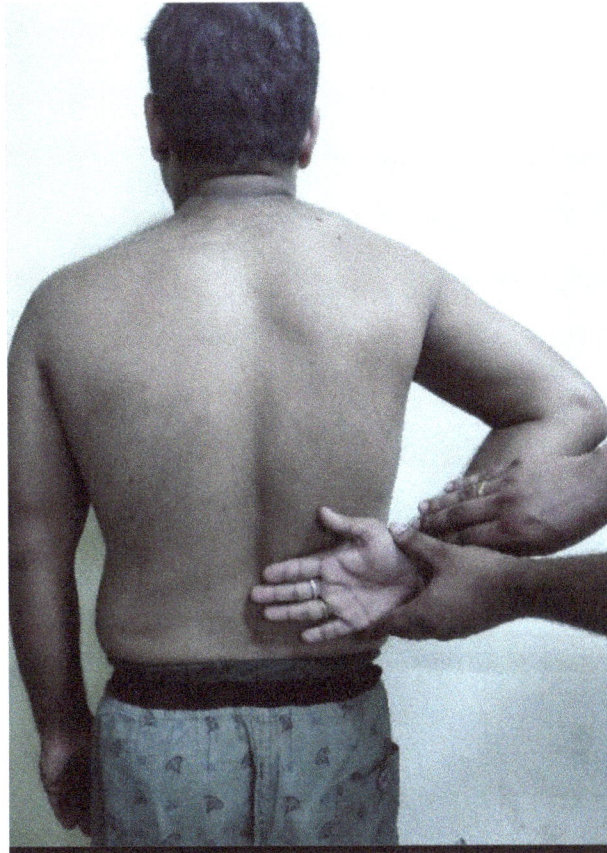

Figure 3. Lift off test.

the arm rotated internally [10].The examiner places hand on the abdomen so he can feel the how much pressure patient is applying. The test is considered positive if the pressing force is weaker or if the pressing movement of the hand against the belly is possible only with the elbow extension and shoulder extended. This indicates a deficiency of the subscapularis tendon tear or dysfunction (**Figure 4**).

The Napoleon test: It is similar to belly press test also called as modified belly press test. The patient hand is placed on abdomen with hand wrist and elbow in straight line. Now patient has to press down on the abdomen negative test indicates wrist at 0° suggestive of normal subscapularis. Positive test indicates patient can press on the belly by flexing wrist at 90° and intermediate result when wrist flexed 30–60° suggestive of partial function of subscapularis. It has sensitivity of 25% and specificity of 97.3%.

The bear-hug test: This test is most sensitive (60%) and with specificity >90%, can be considered single most accurate test for subscapularis injuries [11]. In this test patient has to place his hand on the opposite shoulder with the elbow anterior to the body. The examiner then applies an external rotation force while the patient attempts to maintain the hand on the shoulder. Positive test indicates patient cannot maintain the hand against the shoulder as examiner applies external rotation force (**Figure 5**).

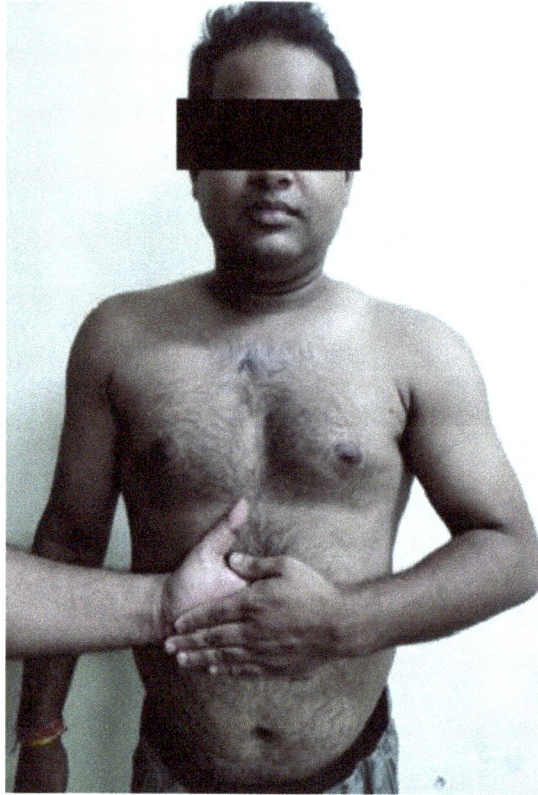

Figure 4. Belly press test.

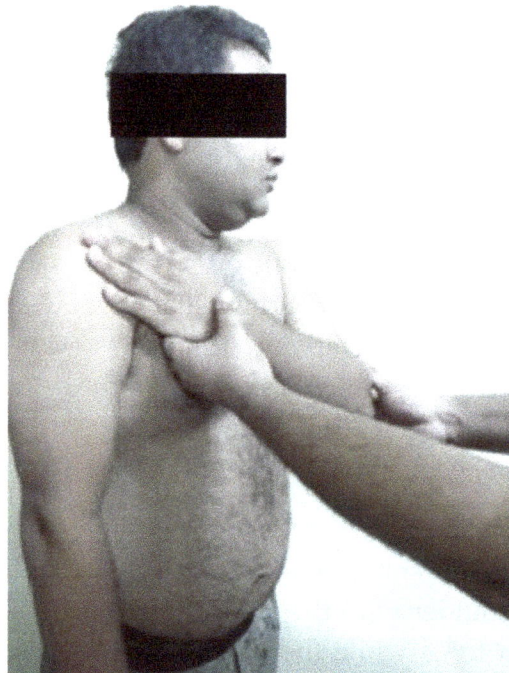

Figure 5. Bear hug test.

All these tests allow diagnosing a partial tear in 30% of cases. More than 50% of tendon thickness is torn when the Napoleon test is positive; more than 75% when the lift-off test is positive.

5. Imaging

X-Rays will demonstrate any coracoid pathology, associated acromial spur degenerative changes (**Figures 6** and **7**).

Ultrasonography (USG) is less reliable than MRI in diagnosing the Subscapularis tears.

USG is more preferred to assess the tendon repaired after shoulder arthroscopy (**Figure 8**).

MRI is the noninvasive procedure of choice to diagnose subscapularis rears. It provides higher diagnostic reliability. Arthro-MRI is even more perfect and accurate as compared to conventional MRI in patients with subscapularis tendon tears.

An indirect sign, often associated with partial subscapularis tears, is a medial dislocation of the long head of the biceps.

There are high chances of partial tears being missed on conventional MRI as compared to Contrast MRI. Fatty degeneration (fatty infiltration) is negative prognostic factor for full

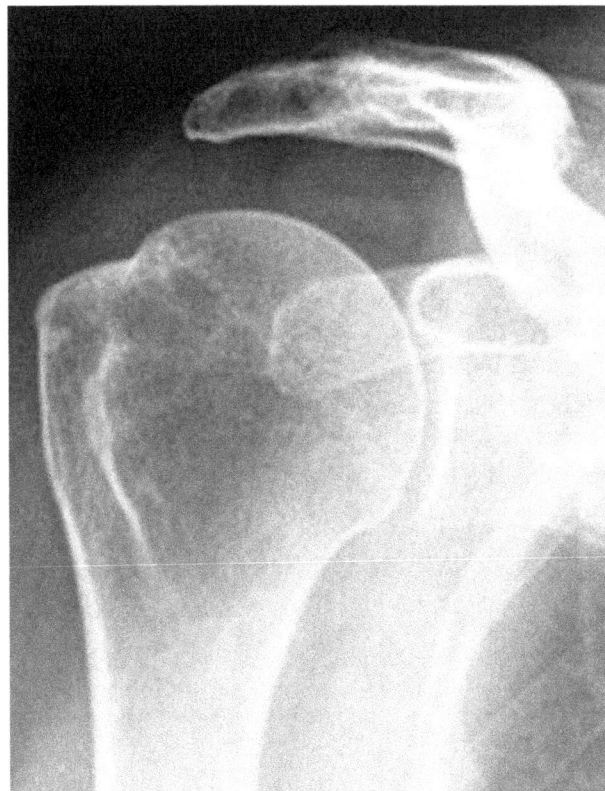

Figure 6. X-ray rockwood view.

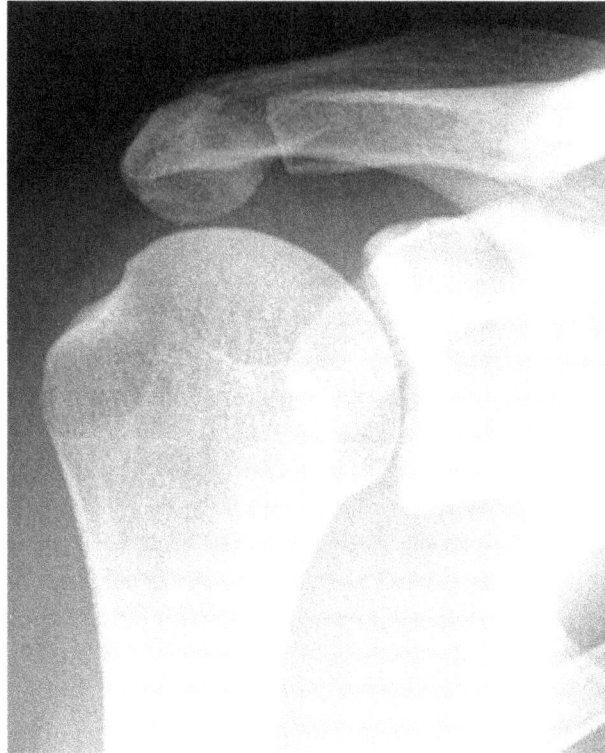

Figure 7. Coracoid impingement x-ray.

functional recovery of the shoulder. The percentage of fatty infiltration predictive of success after cuff repair is lower than 75%.

MR arthrography is accurate in the detection and grading of lesions in the subscapularis tendon. The specificity of findings on transverse images for this diagnosis can be improved by including ancillary signs and findings from parasagittal images (**Figures 9–11**).

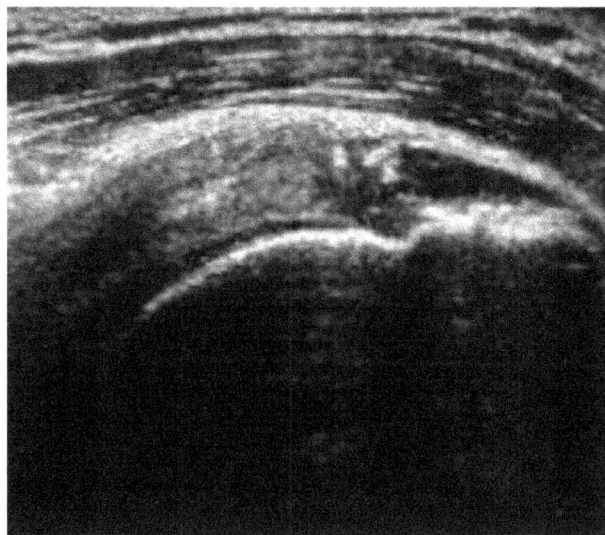

Figure 8. Ultrasonography of subscapularis tear.

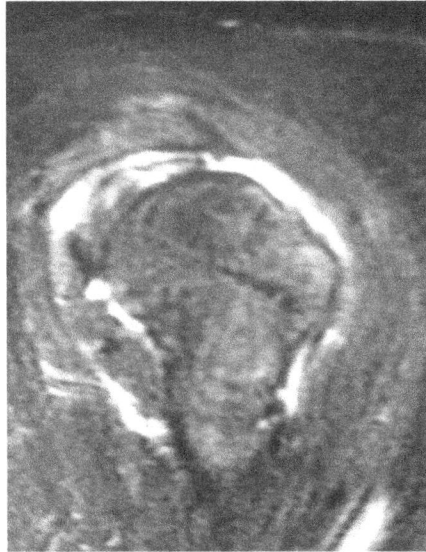

Figure 9. MRI axial view.

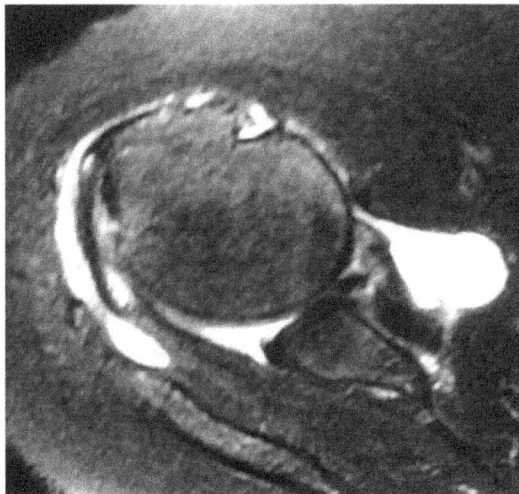

Figure 10. MRI coronal view.

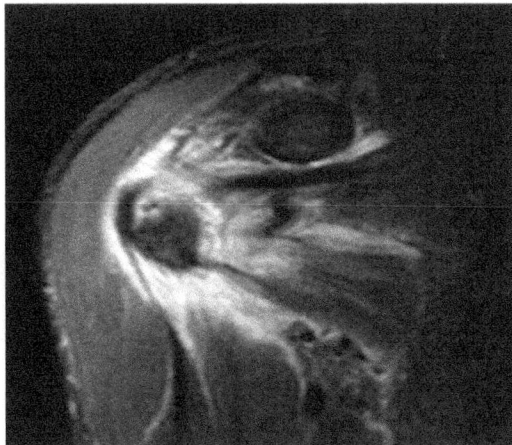

Figure 11. MRI showing rotator cuff muscles.

6. Types of subscapularis tears

In comparison with other rotator cuff tears, subscapularis tear is less common, it seems to have been underestimated. Because of recent attentions to subscapularis tendon, new types of such tendon's lesions have been identified and described. The subscapularis tendon tears may be classified as partial and complete, retracted and not retracted, superior involving the upper third and inferior (extended to the lower third. Lafosse described a five-type classification of subscapularis tendon lesions according to anatomic data and arthroscopic lesion-related findings.

The classification system by Lafosse:

II Complete lesion superior one third

III Complete lesion superior two-thirds

IV Complete lesion with head centered and fatty degeneration<stage3

V Complete lesion with eccentric head and fatty degeneration>stage3

A type I tear is a simple erosion of the upper third of the tendon without any disconnection to the bone (**Figure 12**).

In a type II is a frank detachment of the upper portion of the tendon (**Figure 13**).

A type III lesion is characterized by involvement of all the insertion of the tendon without detachment of the lower third of the muscular portion (**Figure 14**).

In type IV tears, the subscapularis tendon is completely detached from the lesser tuberosity and the humeral head is centered within the joint (**Figure 15**).

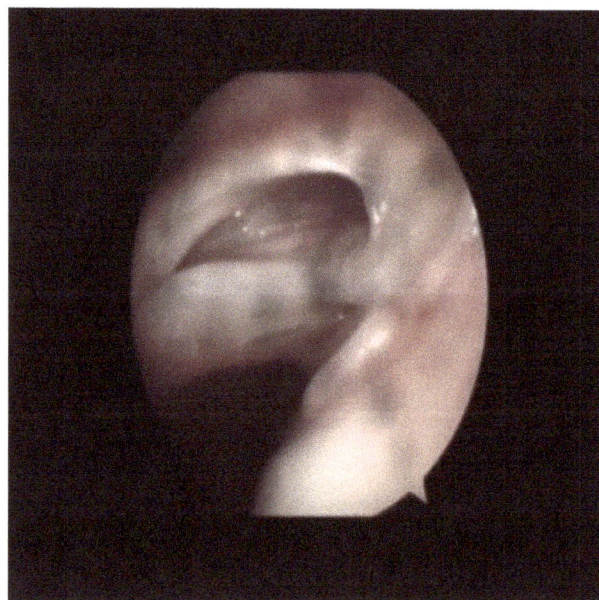

Figure 12. Type I tear.

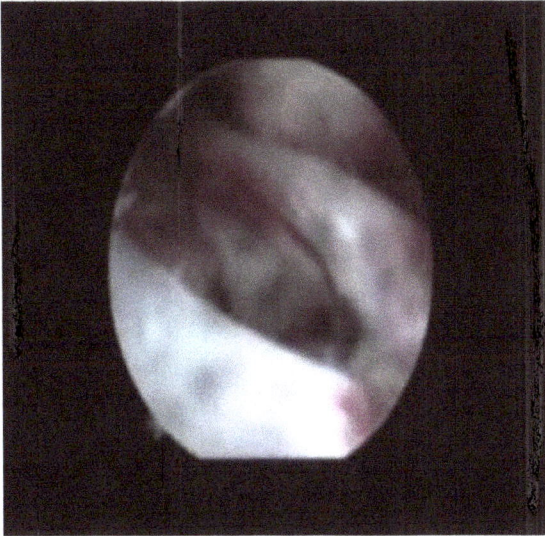

Figure 13. Type II tear.

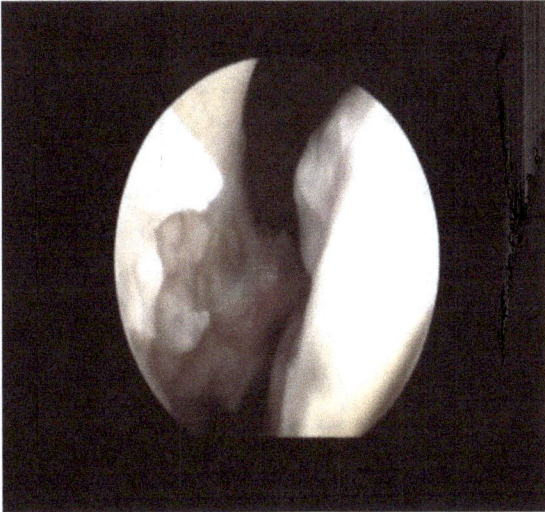

Figure 14. Type III tear.

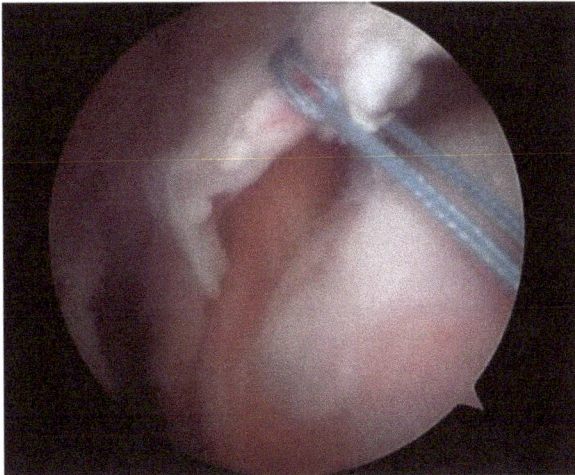

Figure 15. Type IV tear.

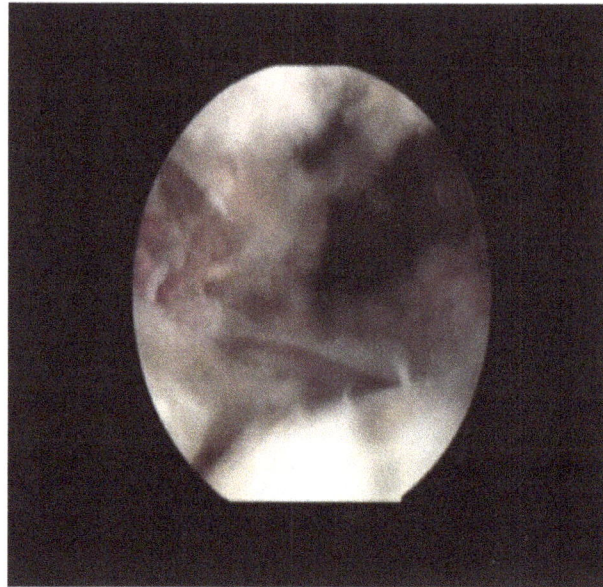

Figure 16. Type V tear.

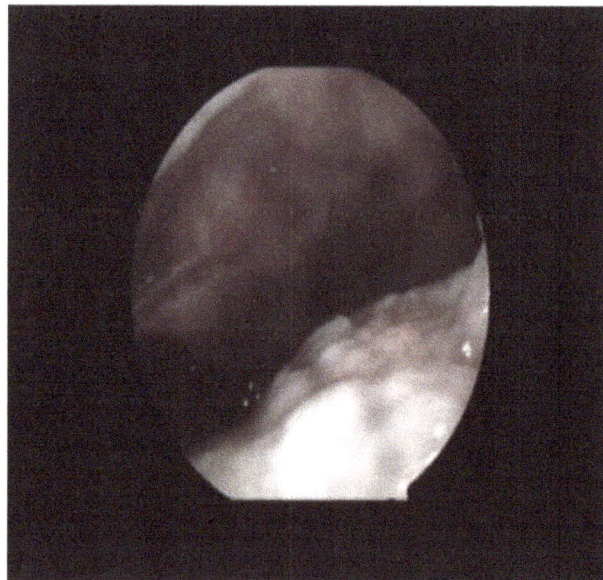

Figure 17. Type V tear Intra-articular view.

In a type V lesion, the lesion is complete, the humeral head is translated anteriorly and superiorly, with coracoid impingement and fatty degeneration of the muscle fibers of the subscapularis (**Figures 16** and **17**).

7. Treatment

There are multiple treatment options in the management of subscapularis tears, with non-operative care indicated in some. In older, inactive patients with smaller a traumatic tears a conservative treatment comprised of physical therapy, anti-inflammatories, and activity modification must be tried. Patients unresponsive to conservative treatment can be considered for surgical repair.

7.1. Open repair

Open repair surgery is performed by deltopectoral approach or anterior deltoid splitting approach in beach chair position. The anterior deltoid splitting approach is mainly used in subscapularis tear associated with supraspinatus or infraspinatus. The deltopectoral approach is used in isolated subscapularis tear. In deltopectoral approach advantage is deltoid is still intact and we can visualize retracted subscapularis tendon. Careful blunt dissection should be done to protect axillary nerve as it lies inferior border of subscapularis. In both approaches we have to open rotator interval from bicipital groove to glenoid. We should be careful for any bicep tendon or supraspinatus pathologies. "Bare bone" will be present between the lesser tuberosity and articular humeral head when there will be complete tear of subscapularis. To visualize the superior subscapular tendon margin, the humeral head must be pushed posteriorly and the tendon seen inside the glenohumeral joint. Tendon should be isolated and then released from its insertion site. In the bare area on the lesser tuberosity with the help of suture anchors or intraosseous sutures the detached tendon is fixed. To fully mobilize the torn tendon if the tendon is too much retracted then release of glenohumeral ligament on the articular side

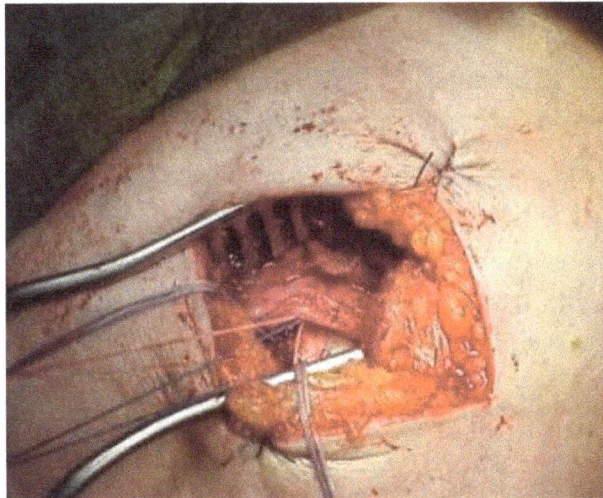

Figure 18. Open subscap tear.

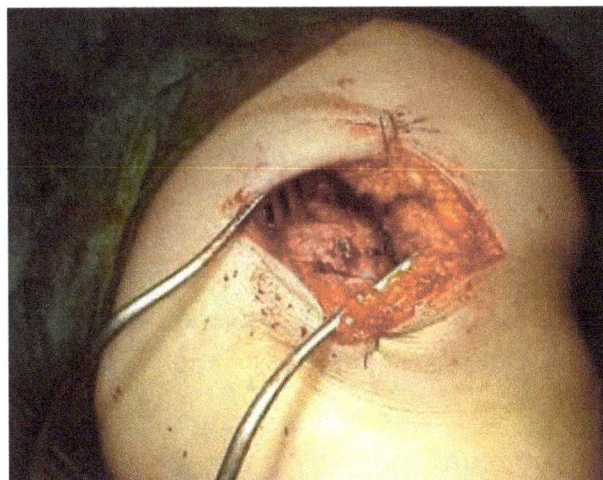

Figure 19. Open repair.

becomes very important step. Once the surgery is complete, the surgeon must assess the range of motion of the shoulder as well as the stability of the repair (**Figures 18** and **19**).

8. Arthroscopic repair

Arthroscopic subscapularis repair surgery can be done with the patient in lateral or beach-chair position. Arthroscopy allows a complete visualization of intraarticular aspects of the joint. In proper position the subscapularis footprint can be visualized that is arm in abduction and internal rotation. For improved visualization of the footprint, a new technique described by Burkhart that is "Posterior lever push." In this technique, the elbow is grasped while a posterior force is applied on the humerus. This results into better visualization of subscapularis insertion site as the intact fibers are pulled away from footprint. This technique may increase the field of view by 5–10 mm. Another method is use of a 70° scope for better visualization of the footprint. The assessment of the tear depends upon the size, direction of the tear and the amount of retraction. It becomes highly impossible to distinguish from conjoint tendon when the tendon is totally retracted. In this situation, finding of "the comma sign," an arc-shaped area of tissue at the superior-most aspect of the subscapularis becomes important. Fibers from the superior glenohumeral ligament as well as the medial head of the coracohumeral ligament comprise the "comma" which serves as a useful lighthouse for the tendon edge.

Biceps tendon pathology like medial subluxation, tears and even SLAP lesions are common with Subscapularis tears, it should be evaluated. The biceps tenotomy or tenodesis is required in order to enhance visualization and protect the repair in case of these pathologies. After a tear of the subscapularis has been identified, subsequent repair should be performed before other shoulder areas are addressed.

Mainly three portals are made to repair the subscapularis.

The posterior portal (P) is the primary viewing portal as commonly used in glenohumeral arthroscopy.

An anterosuperolateral portal (AL) is used to prepare the subscapularis footprint as well as for repair. It lies just anterior to the biceps tendon and anterolateral edge of the acromion.

An anterior portal (AI), is made on just lateral to the coracoid process and it is used for anchor placement.

It becomes very difficult to treat retracted subscapularis tears due to inadequate immobilization. Lo and Burkhart describe the "interval slide in continuity" in which part of the rotator interval and coracohumeral ligament are resected and released in order to increase mobility of the subscapularis tendon. The coracohumeral ligament is "peeled away" from the lateral coracoid, which provides the subscapularis with greater excursion. Preservation of the coracohumeral ligament also allows stable tissue for any associated posterior tears to be approximated via margin convergence.

In this procedure foot print is made by using the same principles that are used for rotator cuff surgery. When the lesions are retracted the bone surface is carefully decorticated, the foot print and subchondral bone exposure is medialised up to 7 mm. Healing process and biological response at the bone tendon interface is improved by micro fractures [12].

Depending upon choices absorbable or non-absorbable anchor sutures can be used in same manner like rotator cuff repair surgery. In almost all cases single anchor suture can be sufficiently used. It is advised that biomechanically one anchor for each square cm. of bare foot print area. It is advised that double row repair has advantages like in rotator cuff surgery in terms of strength and least failure rates. You can use bridging sutures or knotless anchors alternatively. To pass the sutures we can use same techniques that we are using in rotator cuff surgery, paying attention that the sub-coracoid space is far narrower than the sub-acromial space. By using small instruments which pass within the tendon without damaging lesion further, double layer and splitting tears need to be noted. Diagnostic arthroscopy can be used in partial tears thus allowing to undertake transtendineous repair similarly to repair of "PASTA" lesions of the rotator cuff [13] (**Figures 20–31**).

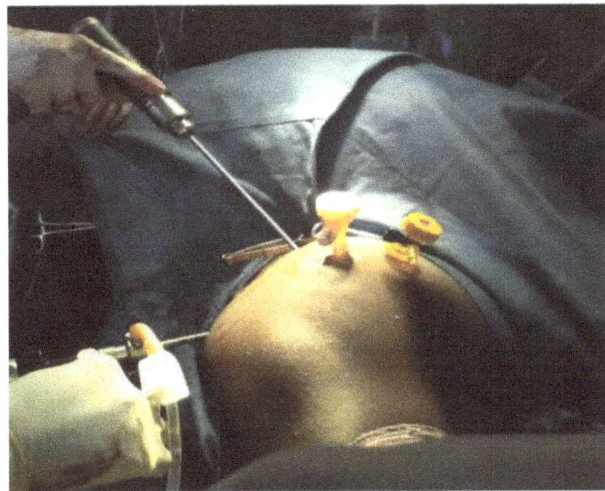

Figure 20. Arthroscopy positions and portals.

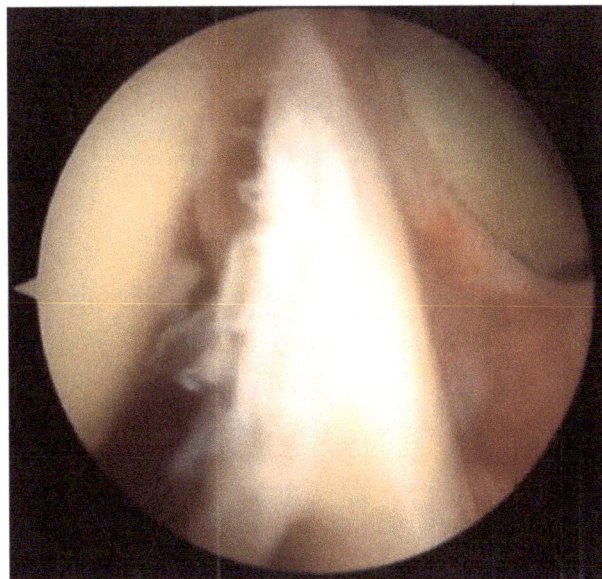

Figure 21. Arthroscopy glenohumeral view.

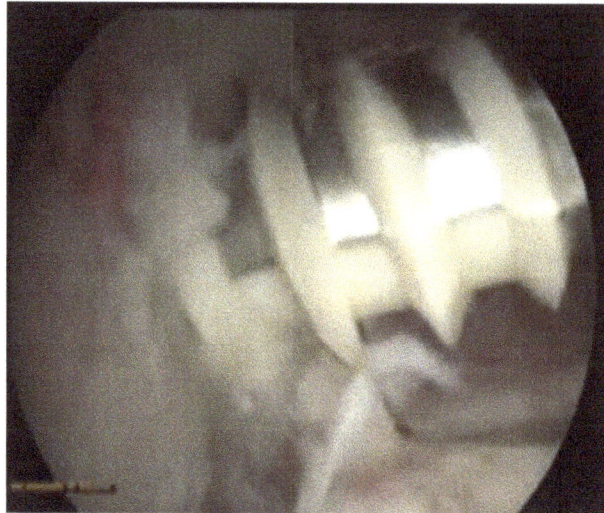

Figure 22. Anchor inserted.

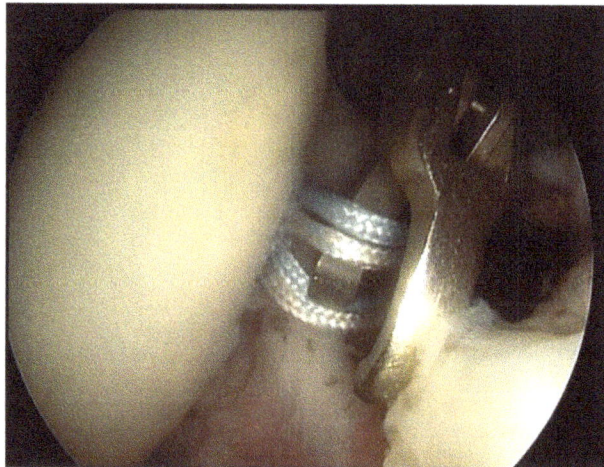

Figure 23. Sutures management.

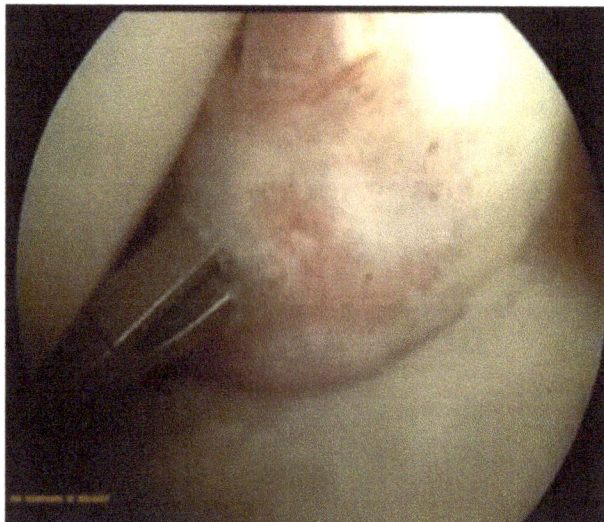

Figure 24. Sutures passing through tendon.

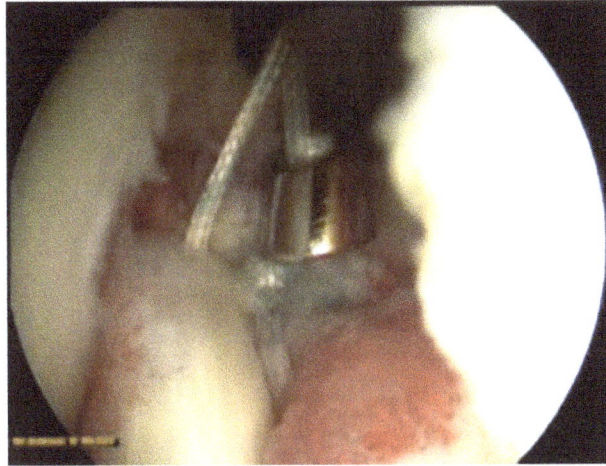

Figure 25. Completed repair.

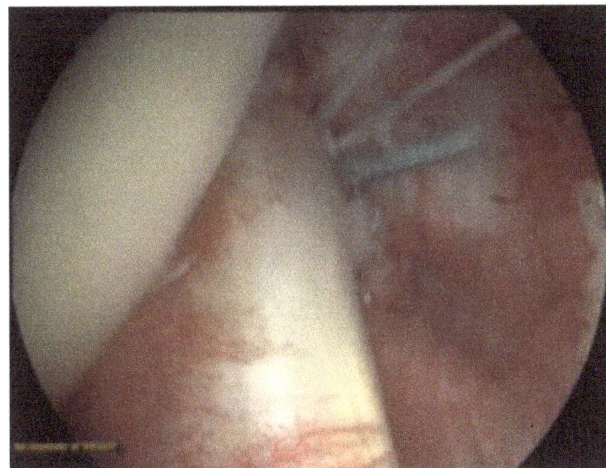

Figure 26. Tout tendon after repair.

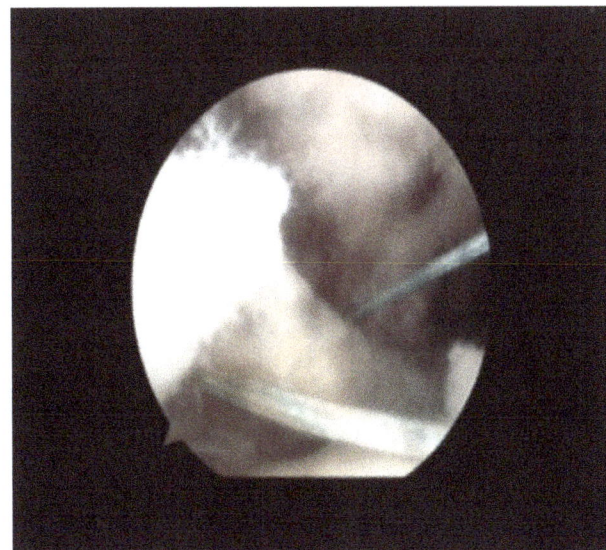

Figure 27. Full thickness tear sub acromial view.

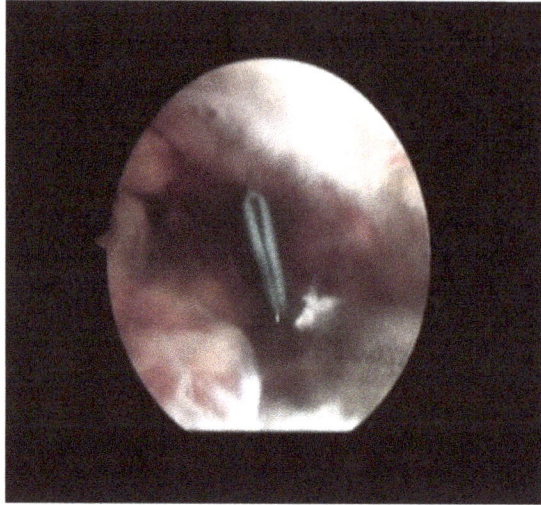

Figure 28. Suture passing through tendon.

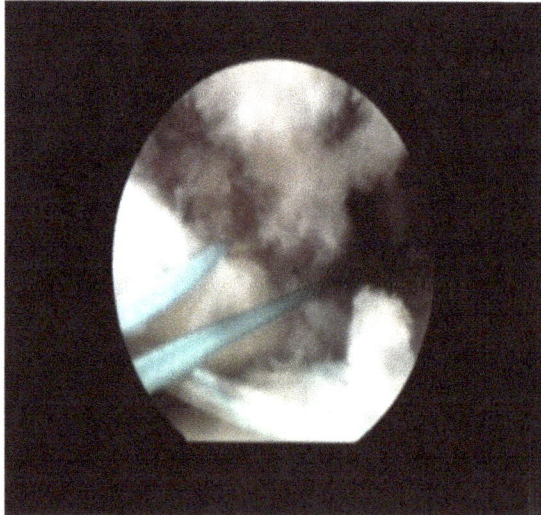

Figure 29. Special instrument for suture passing.

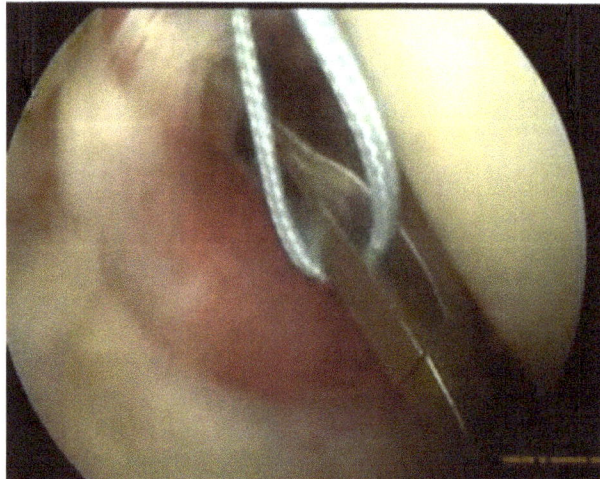

Figure 30. Suture management.

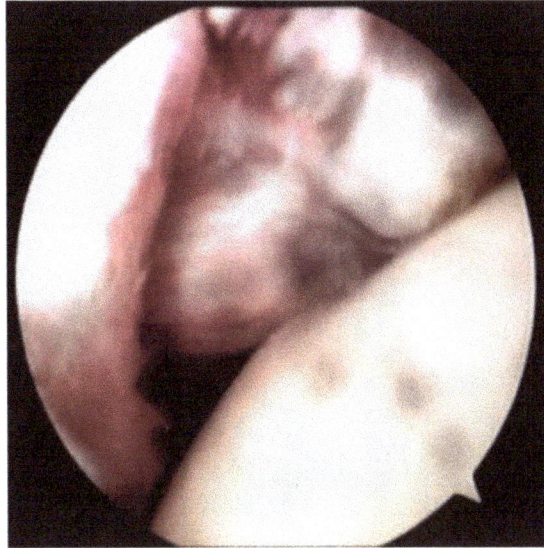

Figure 31. Final repair.

9. Rehabilitation

Physiotherapy protocol is usually individualized as per the Type of tear, Bone and tissue quality, Patients age and physical status and involvement of other Cuff muscles.

Day 0–Day 21:

- Arm pouch.
- Passive ROM as tolerated except external rotation and extension.
- Scapular retraction and rear deltoid exercises.

4th–6 week:

- Gradual full ROM.
- Start active assisted exercises.
- Arm pouch during travel and sleep.

7th–12 weeks:

- No sling.
- Start normal activities.
- Active Thera band exercises for rotator cuff and Scapular muscles.

4th–6 months:

- Weight training for deltopectoral and Biceps-Triceps muscles.
- Sports specific training (**Figures 32** and **33**).

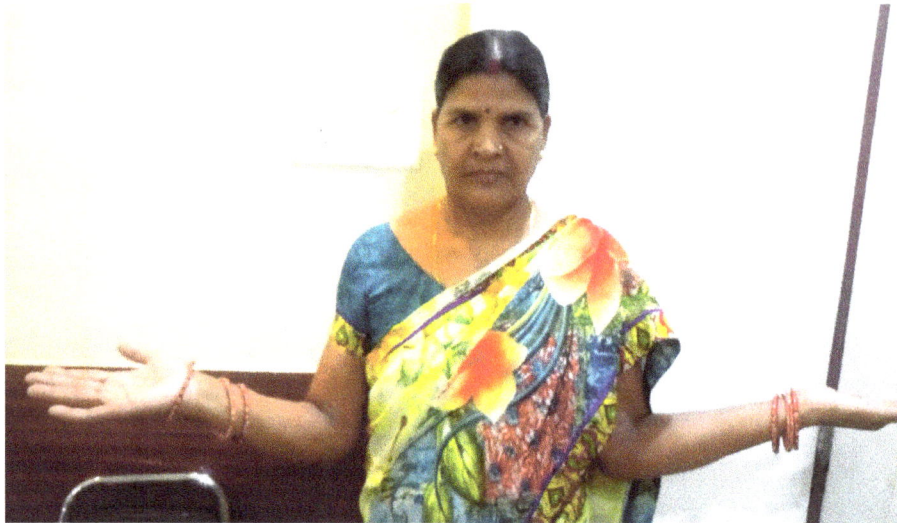

Figure 32. Function post physiotherapy.

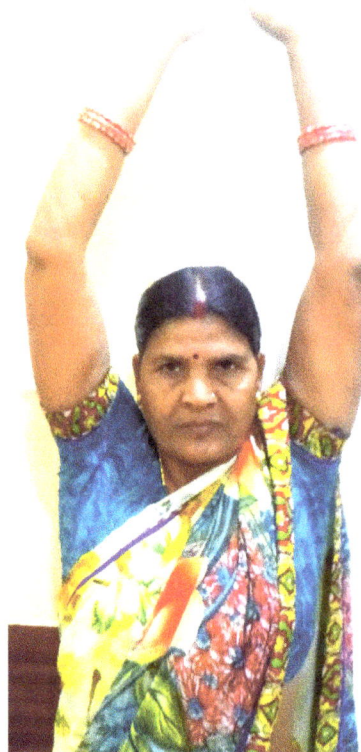

Figure 33. Excellent strength and functions.

Author details

Omkar P. Kulkarni and Satish B. Sonar*

*Address all correspondence to: stshsonar@gmail.com

Dr. PDM Medical College, Amravati, India

References

[1] Smith J. Pathological appearances of seven cases of injury of the shoulder joint, with remarks. London Medical Gazette. 1834;**14**:280

[2] Codman E. Complete rupture of the supraspinatus tendon: Operative treatment with report of two successful cases. Boston Medical Surgery. **20**:708-710

[3] Hauser E. Avulsion of the tendon of the subscapularis muscle. The Journal of Bone and Joint Surgery. American Volume. 1954;**36**:139-141

[4] Kato SFH, Kan I, Yoshida M, Kasama K, Marumo K. Incomplete joint side tear of the subscapularis tendon with a small fragment in an adolescent tennis player: A case report. Sports Medicine Arthroscopy Rehabilitation Therapy and Technology. 2012;**4**:24

[5] Bhalla A, Higashigawa K, McAllister D. Subscapularis tendon rupture in an 8-year-old boy: a case report. American Journal of Orthopedics (Belle Mead, N.J.). 2011;**40**:471-474

[6] Lo IK, Burkhart SS. The comma sign: An arthroscopic guide to the torn subscapularis tendon. Arthroscopy. 2003;**19**:334-337

[7] Denard P, Lädermann A, Burkhart S. Arthroscopic management of subscapularis tears. Sports Medicine and Arthroscopy. 2011;**19**:333-341

[8] Foad A, Wijdicks C. The accuracy of magnetic resonance imaging and magnetic resonance arthrogram versus arthroscopy in the diagnosis of subscapularis tendon injury. Arthroscopy. 2012;**28**:636-641

[9] Barth J, Audebert S, Toussaint B, Charousset C, Godeneche A, Graveleau N, Joudet T, Lefebvre Y, Nove-Josserand L, Petroff E, Solignac N, Scymanski C, Pitermann M, Thelu C. Society FA Diagnosis of subscapularis tendon tears: are available diagnostic tests pertinent for a positive diagnosis? Orthopaedics & Traumatology, Surgery & Research. 2012;**98**:S178-S185

[10] Gerber C, Hersche O, Farron A. Isolated rupture of the subscapularis tendon. The Journal of Bone and Joint Surgery. American Volume. 1996;**78**:1015-1023

[11] Barth J, Burkhart S, De Beer J. The bear-hug test: a new and sensitive test for diagnosing a subscapularis tear. Arthroscopy. 2006;**22**:1076-1084

[12] Lafosse L, Lanz U, Saintmard B, Campens C. Arthroscopic repair of subscapularis tear: Surgical technique and results. Orthopaedics & Traumatology, Surgery & Research. 2010;**96**:S99-108

[13] Osti L, Rizzello G, Panascì M, Denaro V, Maffulli N. Full thickness tears: Retaining the cuff. Sports Medicine and Arthroscopy. 2011;**19**:409-419

8

Surgical Approaches in Shoulder Arthroplasty

Brian W. Sager and Michael Khazzam

Abstract

Shoulder arthroplasty is a complex procedure that is becoming increasingly more utilized throughout the world. Due to the numerous static and dynamic stabilizers of the glenohumeral joint, along with the relative proximity to vital neurovascular structures, great care must be taken to access the joint in a safe and effective manner. To date, there are two well-described approaches utilized in shoulder arthroplasty: the deltopectoral approach and the anterosuperior approach. Both of these approaches are effective in accessing the glenohumeral joint; however, due to their anatomic location, they both have distinct advantages and disadvantages. The aim of this book chapter is to describe the methodology for approaching the glenohumeral joint through each of these approaches, as well as to discuss the advantages and disadvantages of utilizing each. In addition, we aim to discuss the various methodologies for closing these wounds and, briefly, to discuss the other approaches described in the orthopedic literature.

Keywords: shoulder, arthroplasty, approaches, deltopectoral, anterosuperior

1. Introduction

Shoulder arthroplasty is becoming an increasingly popular procedure performed for a variety of problems. It has been utilized with great success for advanced degenerative and traumatic conditions of the shoulder [1–5]. Because the shoulder joint is surrounded by vital structures including muscles, nerves, and blood vessels, great care must be taken to ensure safe but adequate exposure to the glenohumeral joint when performing shoulder arthroplasty. To date, the deltopectoral approach [6] and the anterosuperior lateral approach [7] are the two main approaches that have been well described in the literature for access to the glenohumeral joint for shoulder arthroplasty. Each approach offers distinct advantages and disadvantages with regard to glenoid exposure as well as technical challenges for component implantation. The aim of this chapter is to describe these two different approaches to the glenohumeral joint, the indications for use, and the advantages of each.

2. Positioning and draping

The semirecumbent, or beach-chair position, is the optimum position for open approaches to glenohumeral joint. It allows improved orientation for the surgeon, optimal rotational control of the arm, and allows for gravity traction on both the glenohumeral joint and the subacromial space [8]. It is critical that patient positioning allows for stabilization of the scapula to assure proper glenoid orientation. Additionally, equally important is that the patient is placed in a position on the operating table that allows for extension of the shoulder. Failure to recognize this is one of the most commonly made mistakes that can result in difficulty in exposure for both delivery of the proximal humerus out of the surgical wound and adequate exposure of the glenoid (**Figure 1**).

To begin, the patient should be transferred to the operating table and placed into the supine position for intubation. After successful induction of general anesthesia, the patient should be appropriately positioned on the table while supine in order to allow for the safest and easiest transition to the beach-chair position. While the patient is being elevated into position, the anesthesiologist should maintain cervical support while monitoring the airway. The head support should then be elevated to fit the patient's occiput and secured in place. Care must be taken to ensure that the patient's cervical spine remains in a neutral position as anesthesia literature has shown evidence of cerebrovascular and airway incidents that are felt to be caused by inappropriate cervical positioning and subsequent kinking of the carotid artery or trachea [9, 10]. The head should then be secured to the head support in a secure fashion and the endotracheal

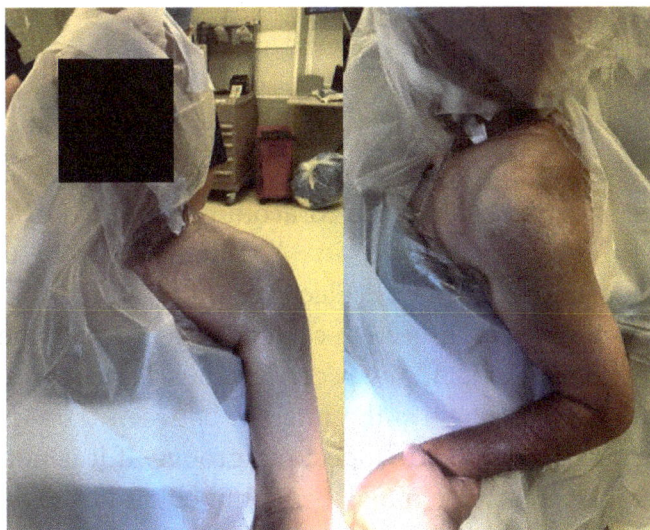

Figure 1. Appropriate positioning and preparation of the shoulder. Please note that the operative shoulder is placed off the edge of the table to allow for extension of the shoulder during the procedure.

tube should be positioned toward the nonoperative side. A pre-scrub with chlorhexidine, alcohol, and/or hydrogen peroxide may then be performed. Finally, a sterile skin preparation with chlorhexidine may be applied prior to final draping. The final draping should consist of down sheets to cover the head and lower extremities with split drapes or a specialized shoulder drape may be used to isolate the operative shoulder. The distal extremity can be placed in a stockinette and covered with a coban wrap, if preferred. An iodine-impregnated plastic drape or any other sterile adhesive dressing may be used to ensure that the edges of the drape adhere to the skin, ensuring a sterile field through the duration of the case. Prior to skin incision, it is important to administer appropriate antibiotics. Typically, this involves a second-generation cephalosporin such as cefazolin or, if the patient has an allergy to penicillin, clindamycin may be substituted. If preoperative testing indicates that the patient is colonized with methicillin-resistant *Staphylococcus aureus* (MRSA), studies show an increased risk of surgical-site infection [11]. In these situations, it is recommended either to decolonize the patient before the surgery or to give a one-time dose of vancomycin [12]. In addition to antibiotics, pre-incision intravenous administration of tranexamic acid has been shown in multiple studies to decrease intraoperative blood loss [13, 14]. At this point, skin incision is ready to be made.

3. Deltopectoral approach

The deltopectoral approach is an anterior approach to the shoulder that utilizes the plane between the deltoid and the pectoralis major muscles. It utilizes an internervous plane between the axillary nerve and the medial and lateral pectoral nerves. It is a robust approach to the shoulder as it has been used for fixation of proximal humerus fractures, reconstruction for shoulder instability, access to the glenohumeral joint in the setting of a septic shoulder, and others [15, 16]. When accessing the glenohumeral joint from the deltopectoral approach, the subscapularis tendon lies directly anterior to the joint capsule. It must be released to access the joint and there are a variety of methods for doing so which will be described in this chapter [17–19].

3.1. Superficial dissection

The surgeon should begin by palpating the bony landmarks around the shoulder, including the acromion, the clavicle, and the coracoid process. An 8–10-cm incision should be marked out, extending from the lateral margin of the coracoid process and extending down the deltopectoral groove toward the deltoid tuberosity. A scalpel should be used to carry the incision through the skin and the dermal layer. Electrocautery can then be used to address any bleeding in the subcutaneous layer. Dissection can continue through the subcutaneous tissue until the fascia overlying the deltoid and the pectoralis muscles is reached. At this point, careful dissection should be used to identify the interval between these muscles. The cephalic vein may be visualized running in the deltopectoral groove. If it is not evident, often times, a stripe of fat overlying the cephalic vein may be identified and used as a helpful marker for identifying the interval (**Figure 2**). The vein should be freed from the surrounding structures and retracted either medially or laterally, depending on surgeon preference. An anatomic study was performed on 40 cadaveric specimens with latex injection of the cephalic vein.

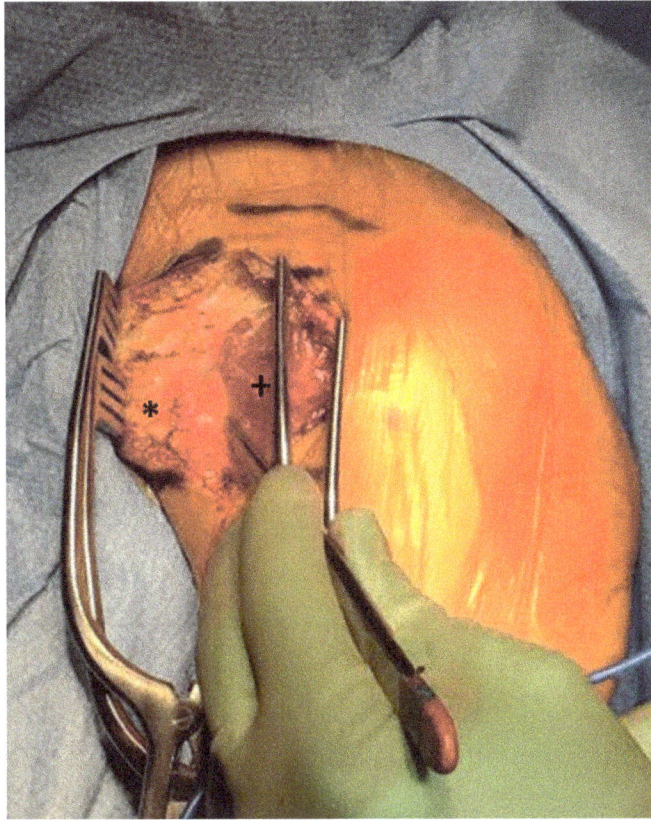

Figure 2. Deltopectoral interval as demarcated by the stripe of fat overlying the cephalic vein. The pectoralis major is identified by the *, while the deltoid is marked by the +.

The authors found more branches from the cephalic vein on the deltoid side, allowing them to conclude that lateral retraction may be more efficacious in preventing bleeding [20]. Once the vein has been retracted, blunt dissection can be used to identify the undersurface of both muscle bellies. A kobel retractor can then be used with one blade under each muscle belly, allowing exposure of the clavipectoral fascia and conjoined tendons of the short head of the biceps and the coracobrachialis (**Figure 3**). Once the fascia is divided in line with the incision, it is pivotal to identify the axillary nerve as it courses near the inferior border of the subscapularis tendon. The surgeon should gently palpate medially over the musculotendinous junction and feel for the axillary nerve. Once found, the nerve should be protected with retractors through the duration of the case. The nerve will then travel posteriorly as it passes inferior to the glenoid where it exits the quadrangular space along with the posterior circumflex humeral vessels. A kobel retractor should be utilized to retract the conjoined tendon medially, exposing the subscapularis tendon over the anterior aspect of the glenohumeral joint. Care must be taken to avoid excessive retraction of the conjoined tendon to avoid a neuropraxia of the musculocutaneous nerve [21].

3.2. Handling of the subscapularis

In order to access the glenohumeral joint capsule, the subscapularis tendon must be mobilized and retracted from the operative field. In the literature, three methods for releasing the

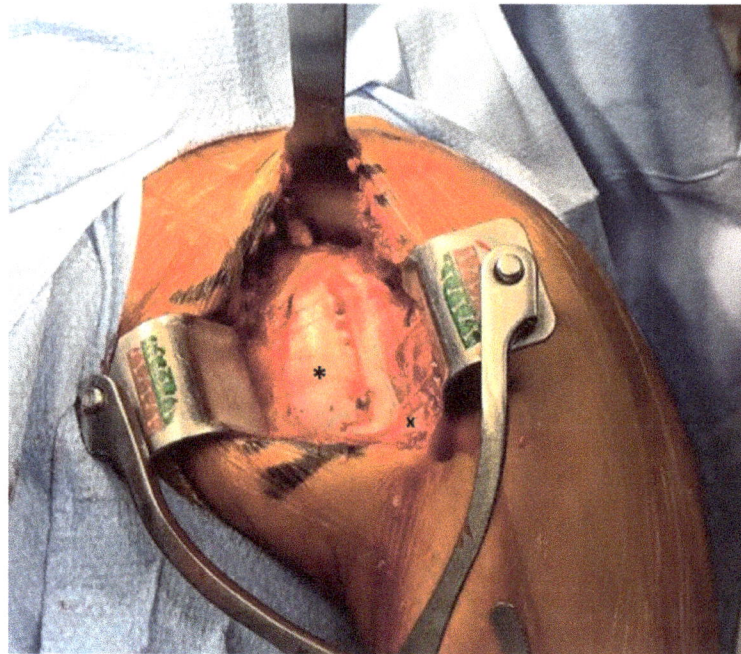

Figure 3. After splitting the deltopectoral interval, the conjoint tendon of the coracobrachialis and the short head of the biceps can be visualized, marked by the *. The pectoralis major tendon is marked with an X.

subscapularis have been described: a tenotomy [19], peeling the tendon off the lesser tuberosity [18], or an osteotomy of the lesser tuberosity [22]. Each of the methods will be described and compared in this chapter. The methods for repair for each of these procedures will be described in the closure section.

3.2.1. Subscapularis tenotomy

When preparing to tenotomize the subscapularis tendon, it is important to identify the superior and inferior borders of the tendon. The arm should be held in adduction and external rotation as it tensions the subscapularis tendon and moves the tenotomy site further away from the axillary nerve. The tenotomy should be made approximately 1 cm medial to the subscapularis insertion on the lesser tuberosity of the humerus. This is typically the location of the anatomic neck of the humerus. It is important to leave a small cuff of subscapularis tendon on the lesser tuberosity to which to repair the tendon during closure. In addition, when releasing the inferior portion of the subscapularis, it is necessary to identify and cauterize the anterior humeral circumflex artery and the two accompanying veins in order to prevent retraction and subsequent bleeding. When performing the tenotomy, it can be helpful to place two large-caliber, braided sutures in the medial aspect of the tendon in order to hold tension during the tenotomy and to help during repair of the tenotomy. When performing a tenotomy for shoulder arthroplasty, the tenotomy and subsequent capsulotomy may be performed simultaneously by releasing the deeper tissues and continuing the dissection along the neck of the humerus. If this method is chosen, it is very important to place a blunt retractor between your dissection and the axillary nerve, coursing inferior to the glenoid, in order to prevent iatrogenic injury (**Figure 4**). Alternatively, the subscapularis may be released

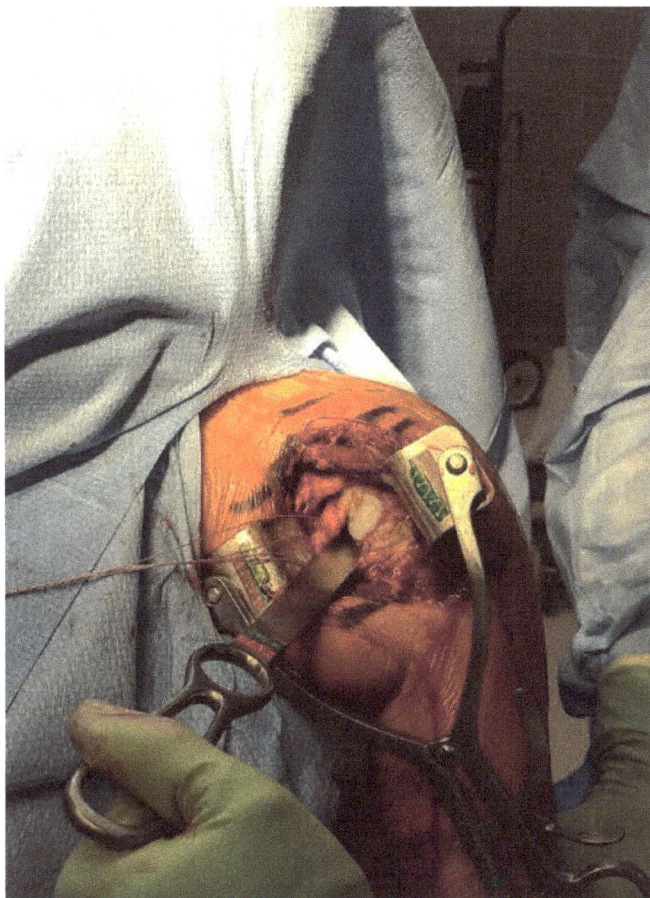

Figure 4. Subscapularis tendon after tenotomy. Note the stay sutures placed in the medial limb of the subscapularis tendon. Also, please note the placement of the Darrach retractor at the inferomedial border of the subscapularis protecting the axillary nerve.

from the anterior capsule prior to arthrotomy, but this method provides less robust tissue for later repair and may lead to subscapularis failure. This approach is the easiest and quickest to perform and repair of all the listed methods. It has been associated with good long-term outcomes [23]. While tendon-to-tendon healing is a reliable means of healing, data in the literature are mixed in regard to maintenance of subscapularis repair with some studies showing excellent healing rates [24] and others showing attenuation or ruptures being common [25]. One disadvantage to this method is the inability to medialize the insertion of the subscapularis tendon or the potential for shortening the tendon during repair causing limits in postoperative external rotation.

3.2.2. Subscapularis peel

Another method of releasing the subscapularis tendon is the subscapularis peel. Rather than releasing the tendon through a division within the substance of the tendon, the subscapularis is elevated in its entirety off of its insertion on the lesser tuberosity. After the subscapularis has been released from the lesser tuberosity, dissection should proceed as described earlier. The major advantage of the subscapularis peel is that it allows for medialization of the insertion of the subscapularis tendon [26]. In addition, peeling the subscapularis off the humerus will allow for maximal surface area for bony healing to occur. The biggest drawback of this procedure is the need for tendon-to-bone healing to occur in order to maintain subscapularis function, which is, generally, felt to be less reliable than tendon-to-tendon or bone-to-bone. However, the literature does vary as there are studies showing excellent healing rates in patients undergoing a subscapularis peel [27]. In addition, the repair requires violating the cortex, thus weakening the proximal humerus.

3.2.3. Lesser tuberosity osteotomy

Lastly, the insertion of the subscapularis tendon, the lesser tuberosity, may be osteotomized and retracted without disrupting the tendon itself. Initially, the long head of the biceps tendon can be released and subsequently tenodesed to the upper margin of the pectoralis major tendon. Once the biceps tendon is out of the way, the lesser tuberosity may be visualized in its entirety. The arm should be held in adduction and internal rotation and an osteotome or oscillating saw should be used to perform the osteotomy from the medial aspect of the bicipital groove to the bone-cartilage interface at the anatomic neck. After the lesser tuberosity has been osteomized, freeing the remainder of the subscapularis should proceed as described in the tenotomy section. The lesser tuberosity osteotomy was originally introduced to provide a method of repairing the subscapularis which relied on bone-to-bone healing and did not violate the tendon itself. Healing rates have been shown to be excellent for this method [17, 22]. In addition, medialization of the tendon remains possible with this procedure. The disadvantages of this procedure include difficulty and timeliness of procedure, as well as the potential for iatrogenic fracture or nonunion due to violation of the cortical bone.

3.2.4. Comparisons

There have been several studies in the literature comparing the outcomes, biomechanics, and healing potential of the subscapularis tendon after the above procedures [25, 27–30]. Two cadaver biomechanical studies evaluated the failure rates of the above three methods of repair. One showed improved failure rates for both the subscapularis tenotomy and lesser tuberosity osteotomy [29]. Another showed no significant difference between the three methods [30]. Similarly, a biomechanical study comparing lesser tuberosity osteotomy to tenotomy showed no significant difference in load to failure; however, it did show that the tenotomy group had less displacement during repetitive loading [28]. Clinical comparisons between the groups also have mixed outcomes. A randomized controlled trial comparing subscapularis strength and functional outcomes between lesser tuberosity osteotomy versus subscapularis peel showed no significant difference at 2 years [27]. On the contrary, a retrospective study comparing lesser tuberosity osteotomy versus subscapularis tenotomy at an average of 33 months showed improved clinical outcomes and lower rates of subscapularis tears in the osteotomy group [25]. Because of the large amount of conflicting literature, it is likely that the most important factor regarding handling of the subscapularis is surgeon preference and experience. Great care should be taken to ensure an adequate repair while maintaining appropriate tendon length.

3.3. Humeral exposure

As stated earlier, when exposing the humerus after a subscapularis tenotomy, the subscapularis tendon and anterior shoulder capsule may be released as a single unit. However, when performing a subscapularis peel or a lesser tuberosity osteotomy, the subscapularis must be separated from the anterior capsule. This may be done by placing a blunt elevator between the two structures and then using a 15 blade to complete the dissection. Once the capsule has been isolated from the subscapularis, a retractor should be placed at the inferior margin of the glenoid to protect the axillary nerve. A capsulotomy may then be performed with sharp dissection or electrocautery extending along the anatomic neck of the humerus, continuing inferior down the humerus. It is important to dissect along the humerus to avoid damaging the nearby neurovascular structures. It is critical to release the capsule off of the neck of the humerus until the latissimus dorsi tendon is visualized as it wraps around the humerus. This provides not only assurance that complete visualization of the anatomic neck of the humerus and accompanying osteophytes is attained but also aids in glenoid visualization. The exposed osteophytes around the humerus should then be removed using a rongeur. Once the humerus has been exposed, a deltoid retractor can be placed posterior to the head to facilitate exposure of the head. The arm should be adducted, extended, and externally rotated in order to dislocate the head and deliver it into the surgical site (**Figure 5**). A Hohmann retractor may be placed on the calcar and a Darrach should be placed medially to protect the soft tissues, specifically the rotator cuff, during the humeral head cut. Depending on the implant system being utilized, an intramedullary or extramedullary cutting guide may be used to help guide your humeral head cut. If performing the cut freehand, the cut should be made along the anatomic neck of the humerus with care taken to avoid violating the supraspinatus insertion on the greater tuberosity. The angle of the cut should match the neck-shaft angle of the implant if the implant is a fixed angle device. Most implants will have a head-neck angle of around 130–140° [31]. After resection, the head should not be removed from the field as it may be useful in deciding implant size and can be used as a source of bone graft if needed. The timing of humeral head resection is typically dictated by surgeon preference and implant system constraints.

3.4. Glenoid exposure

After the humeral head has been cut, a Fukuda, or a Bankart, retractor should be placed on the posterior glenoid neck and used to retract the humeral shaft posteriorly and inferiorly, out of the operative field. A double-pronged retractor can be placed on the anterior glenoid neck, and most importantly a Hohmann or a Darrach retractor can be placed along the inferior glenoid neck to protect the axillary nerve at all times during the glenoid preparation. Anatomic studies have shown that the axillary nerve can range from 3 to 7 mm inferior to the musculotendinous junction of the subscapularis muscle [32, 33]. After appropriate retractors have been placed, electrocautery or a sharp 15 blade may be used to circumferentially remove the subscapularis, capsule, and labrum to expose the entire periphery of the glenoid. A 360 release of the subscapularis must be performed in order to adequately expose the glenoid. The inferior capsule must be released, carefully protecting the axillary nerve. The dissection should continue down the humeral shaft to the level of the latissimus dorsi. Afterwards, a pair of curved Mayo scissors may be used to release the rotator interval superiorly. This should extend to the level of

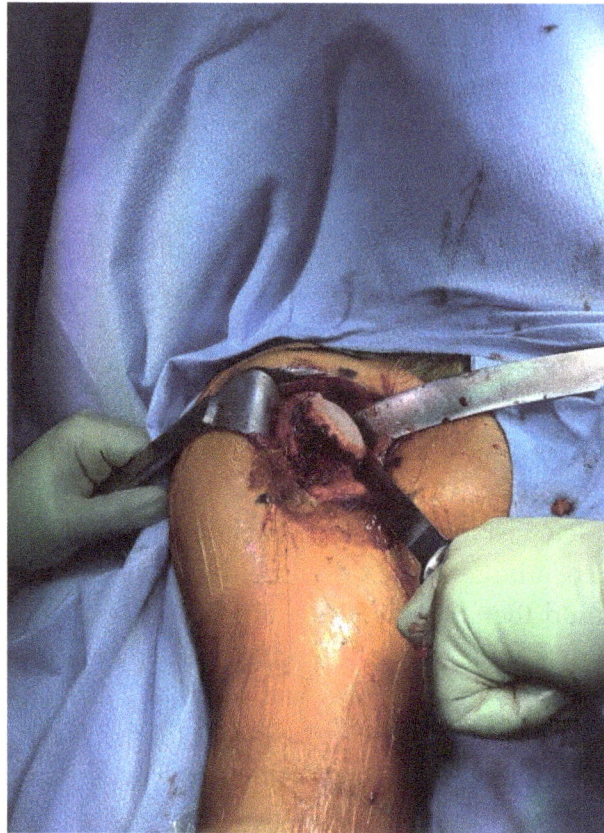

Figure 5. Proximal humeral exposure. The marginal osteophytes have been removed from the subchondral surface using a rongeur. The neck cut should be made along the anatomic neck.

the coracoid base. The anterior capsule should then be dissected from the anterior glenoid with great care taken not to violate the subscapularis tendon (**Figure 6**). Care should be taken to avoid releasing the glenoid capsule beyond the 6 o'clock position due to concerns of posterior instability. If the posterior capsule must be released, it should occur on the humeral side.

3.5. Preparation for implantation

At this point, the humerus and glenoid are exposed and ready to be prepared according to the specific methodology for the desired implant being utilized. As a rule, a guide pin is placed at approximately 11–12 mm above the inferior glenoid rim. This allows for ideal placement of the glenoid component and allows for minimization of scapular notching [34]. Hand reamers are then placed over this guide pin to concentrically ream the glenoid. A drill is then utilized to create a slot in the glenoid for which to place the central peg of the glenoid baseplate. If necessary, screws may be placed around the baseplate. Attention is then turned toward the humerus where the intramedullary canal is found. Sequential reamers are introduced into the humeral canal until adequate fit and fill is achieved. The reamer is removed and serial broaches are introduced until the appropriate size is reached. Trial components may be placed at this time to ensure appropriate range of motion with adequate stability. After implantation of the desired components, the shoulder should again be taken through a range of motion to ensure that the implant is not overstuffed, but also sufficiently stable.

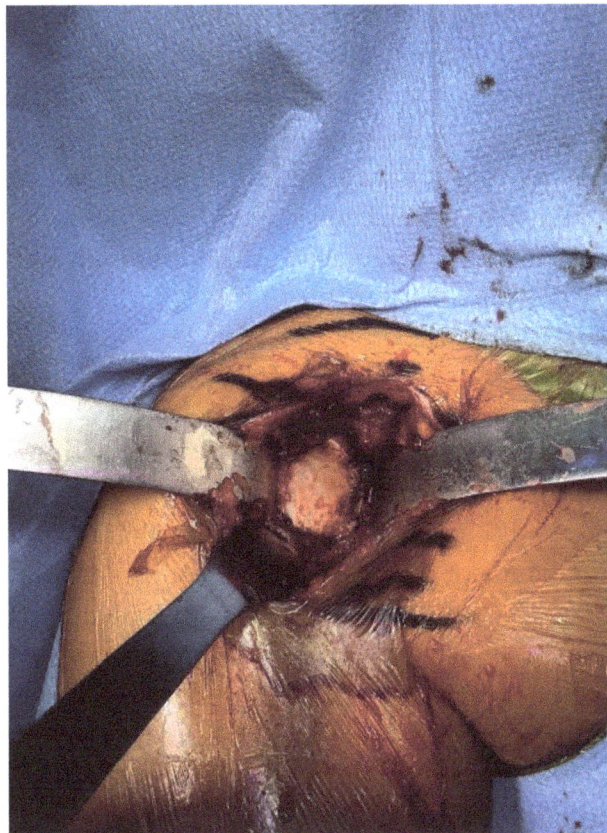

Figure 6. Glenoid exposure. Capsular attachments removed circumferentially around the glenoid.

3.6. Closure

After the components have been appropriately placed and trialed, the wound is ready to be closed. The wound should be irrigated with normal saline. If a significant amount of bleeding was encountered during the surgery, a drain may be placed at this time, if desired. If repairable, the first structure to be repaired is the subscapularis tendon. Depending on how the tendon was released when approaching the shoulder will dictate the method of repair for the tendon. If the subscapularis tenotomy was used, at least three figure-of-eight, large-caliber, braided sutures should be utilized to anatomically repair the tendon. In this particular repair, care should be taken to avoid shortening the tendon as this will result in decreased external rotation function when healed. If the subscapularis was peeled off the lesser tuberosity, the tendon must be repaired using bone tunnels extending from the anatomic neck of the humerus to the lesser tuberosity. Again, heavy, braided, non-absorbable suture should be passed through these drill holes and the subscapularis tendon and tied down in a secure fashion. If the glenohumeral offset was substantially medialized during the procedure, the repair of the insertion of the tendon may be moved more medially to facilitate this. Lastly, if the lesser tuberosity was osteotomized, the surgeon should drill holes in the medial aspect of the bicipital groove. Heavy non-absorbable suture should then be passed around the lesser tuberosity and into the subscapularis tendon. After the lesser tuberosity has been anatomically positioned, it may be secured in place with transosseous sutures. A plate may be placed to augment the repair depending on the preference of the surgeon [26].

After the subscapularis has been securely repaired, the deltopectoral interval may be loosely closed with a running interlocking non-absorbable suture to help identify the interval in future exposure. The subcutaneous layer may be closed in a simple interrupted fashion with either a braided or an unbraided suture depending on surgeon preference. Similarly, the skin may be closed with nylon suture, a running monofilament, staples, or any other acceptable method of skin closure. At this point, a dry dressing or an incisional vacuum should be placed over the wound and the patient should be placed into a sling with an abduction pillow to help keep the arm protected.

3.7. Advantages

The deltopectoral approach is the most commonly used approach to the shoulder-for-shoulder arthroplasty. This is in large part due to the many advantages provided by this approach. This approach is an internervous and intermuscular plane, that is, it utilizes the plane between the deltoid and the pectoralis major muscles. This is important as it preserves the origin of the deltoid and the pectoralis and allows for access beyond the muscles while minimizing the risk of denervation. Furthermore, because the approach is between muscles and not splitting the muscles, less bleeding is observed with this approach. Furthermore, should a fracture arise distal to the stem of the humeral component, it is quite easy to extend the deltopectoral approach into the anterolateral approach to the humerus, utilizing the interval between the brachialis and the brachioradialis. Lastly, approaching the glenohumeral joint from the front allows for easier access to the inferior structures, including the inferior humeral osteophytes and the inferior capsule [35]. Positioning of the glenoid component is also easier with this approach as the inferior portion of the glenoid is more readily available.

3.8. Disadvantages

Though the literature is inconsistent on the matter, many studies have shown that subscapularis-deficient shoulder arthroplasties have higher rates of instability [36, 37]. The deltopectoral approach to the shoulder requires the release of the subscapularis tendon with subsequent repair; however, it is not uncommon for these repairs to fail, leading to a risk of instability in these patients [24, 38]. Furthermore, approaching the glenohumeral joint from the anterior aspect causes difficulty reaching the more posterior structures including the glenoid, capsule, and greater tuberosity. This could be particularly noticeable when performing shoulder arthroplasty for proximal humerus fractures that include a large greater tuberosity fragment. Lynch et al. found that utilizing the deltopectoral approach was an independent risk factor for neurologic complications in total shoulder arthroplasty [39].

4. Anterosuperior approach

The anterosuperior approach to the shoulder was first described by Mackenzie in 1993 [40]. It does not utilize an internervous plane as it requires detachment of the anterior deltoid off the acromion as well as release of the coracoacromial ligament to reach the glenohumeral joint. Though it was initially designed to provide increased exposure of the glenoid for shoulder arthroplasty, it is also frequently used in the open repair of difficult-to-manage rotator-cuff tears [41], proximal humerus fractures, and even long head of the biceps repair. The previously described protocol for anesthesia induction, positioning, and prepping should be utilized for the anterosuperior approach just as it was for the deltopectoral approach.

4.1. Superficial dissection

After the operative arm has been draped, the surgery should begin with the surgeon palpating the bony landmarks of the shoulder including the anterior and posterior aspects of the acromion, as well as the anterior border of the clavicle and the acromioclavicular joint. An approximately 5–7-cm incision should be drawn on the shoulder in line with the longitudinal axis of the clavicle (**Figure 7**). The incision should start just posterior to the anterolateral corner of the acromion and should be carried down through the skin and the subcutaneous tissue until the fascia overlying the deltoid muscle is reached. Careful hemostasis should be achieved with electrocautery. The surgeon should then identify the raphe between the anterior and middle portions of the deltoid (**Figure 8**). Once identified, the raphe should be split in line with the deltoid fibers for approximately 5 cm from the lateral border of the acromion. Care should be taken not to extend the incision beyond 5 cm from the lateral margin of the acromion in order to minimize the risk of damage to the axillary nerve [42]. A stay suture may be placed in the distal aspect of the deltoid to mark the level of the axillary nerve and to help prevent inadvertent damage during dissection. At several instances throughout the course of the surgery, the stay suture should be checked to ensure the integrity of the suture. If it is ever found to be compromised, it should be removed and replaced.

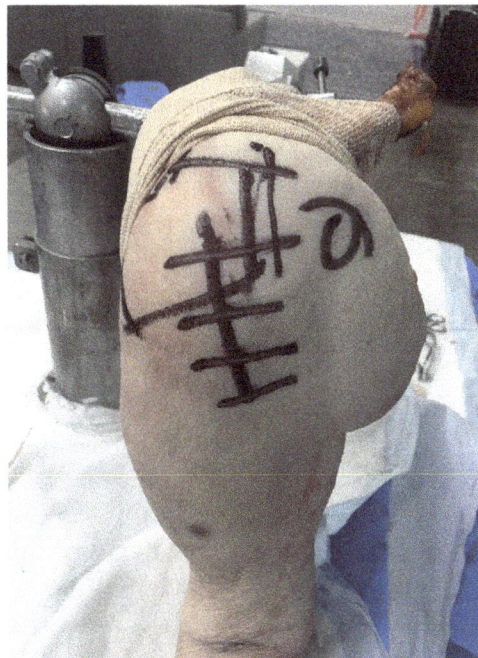

Figure 7. Surface landmarks with incision marked out for the anterosuperior approach. Care should be taken to ensure that the incision is not carried out more than 5 cm below the edge of the acromion to avoid iatrogenic axillary nerve injury. This is a Right shoulder cadeveric specimen.

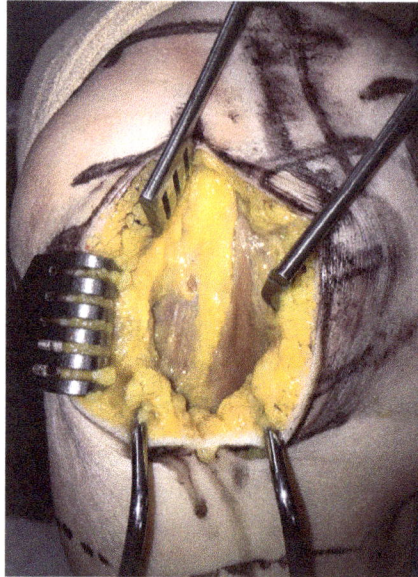

Figure 8. Fat stripe identifying the raphe between the anterior and middle portions of the deltoid.

4.2. Deltoid and coracoacromial ligament handling

At this point, the deltoid separates the surgeon from accessing the glenohumeral joint. The anterosuperior approach to the shoulder mandates the removal of a portion of the deltoid off of the acromion. There are two methods for releasing the anterior deltoid that have been described in the literature. These two methods, acromial osteotomy versus deltoid peel, will be described in this section.

4.2.1. Deltoid peel

The original article by Mackenzie advocated for the removal of approximately 1–2 cm of the deltoid from its origin on the anterior acromion [40]. The deltoid should be reflected in a subperiosteal fashion and care should be taken not to remove more than 2 cm of the deltoid off of the acromion as repairing the deltoid back to the acromion can be difficult. After the deltoid has been retracted out of the way, an acromioplasty of the anterior acromion may be performed to facilitate exposure to the proximal humerus [43]. The coracoacromial ligament may be removed from the undersurface of the acromion using sharp dissection or electrocautery. The acromial branch of the thoracoacromial artery may be encountered deep to the deltoid and should be ligated to prevent retraction and excess bleeding. The subdeltoid bursa can be divided at this time and the long head of the biceps may be identified and then tenotomized at its origin. Peeling the tendon from the acromion requires soft tissue-to-bone healing; however, one recent study showed no changes in axillary nerve or deltoid function 3 months after suture repair of the deltoid back to the acromion [44].

4.2.2. Acromial osteotomy

Rather than peeling the deltoid off the acromion and relying on muscle-to-bone healing, Mole describes an acromial osteotomy to facilitate healing with more robust bone-to-bone healing [7].

Once the dissection has been carried down to the lateral border of the acromion and the deltoid, an osteotome is used to remove a fleck of acromial bone along with the attached deltoid and coracoacromial ligament. This should be retracted, facilitating access now to the glenohumeral joint. Again, if the acromial branch of the thoracoacromial artery is encountered, it should be ligated. If needed, an acromioplasty should be performed in order to better visualize the humerus in preparation for the humeral osteotomy. The subdeltoid bursa should be incised and long head of the biceps tendon should be identified and released at its origin.

4.3. Humeral exposure

After releasing the deltoid and coracoacromial ligament, the humerus is ready to be osteotomized and prepared for implantation. If any question regarding the competency of the subscapularis, supraspinatus, or infraspinatus exists, they may be assessed at this point. In order to visualize the posterior rotator cuff, the arm should be extended and internally rotated to bring the greater tuberosity into the operative field (**Figure 9**). Originally, Mackenzie described a subscapularis tenotomy to allow for anterior dislocation and osteotomy; however, traditionally, the subscapularis has been preserved in this approach. The humeral head should be delivered by subluxating the head anterosuperiorly and the capsular attachments should be removed along the humeral neck. Care should be taken when removing the capsular attachments to cut toward the bone to minimize the risk of damage to surrounding structures. Once the neck is able to be visualized, the humeral head may be cut along the anatomic neck of the humerus with the assistance of implant-specific cutting guides as needed. Again, the excised head should not be removed from the operative field as it may be useful when determining implant size. Once the neck cut has been made, any osteophytes that are observed may be removed using a rongeur or an osteotome. Posterior and inferior osteophytes may be difficult to reach utilizing this approach.

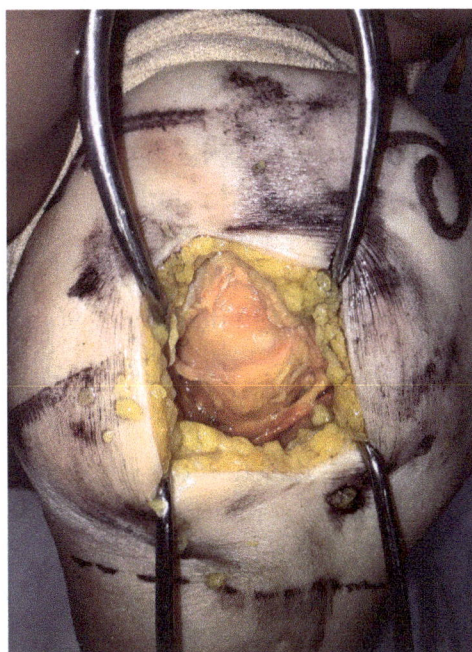

Figure 9. After the deltoid has been peeled off the acromion, the humeral head and rotator-cuff insertion are now visible.

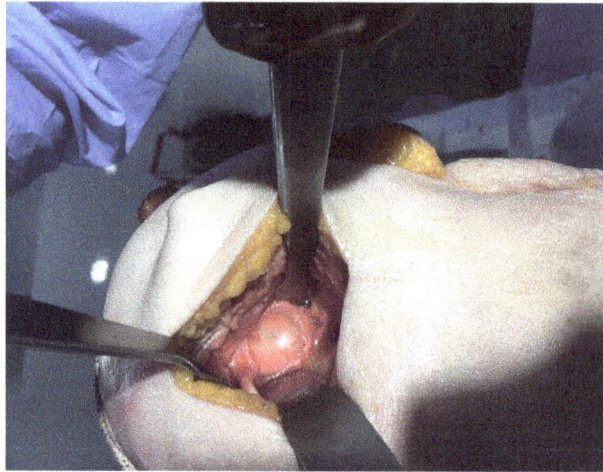

Figure 10. After retraction of the humerus, the anterosuperior approach allows for exceptional glenoid exposure.

4.4. Glenoid exposure

After the humeral neck has been cut, a curved retractor may be placed on the inferior aspect of the glenoid in order to retract the remainder of the humerus posteroinferiorly out of the operative field (**Figure 10**). Another retractor should be placed between the anteroinferior glenoid and the subscapularis tendon in order to protect the axillary nerve as it courses near the undersurface of the glenoid neck. The capsulo-labral attachments should be circumferentially removed from the glenoid periphery using either sharp dissection with a 15 blade or electrocautery.

4.5. Preparation for implantation

Once the humerus and glenoid have been sufficiently exposed, they are ready for preparation. Traditionally, a guide pin is placed in the center aspect of the glenoid in order to establish the axis for the central peg of the glenoid component. Great care should be taken with this particular approach to ensure that adequate inferior tilt of the glenoid component is achieved as the presence of the humerus can significantly interfere with the coronal position of the implant. After the appropriate plane has been achieved, the glenoid is reamed and prepared according to the implant-specific methods. The glenoid component should then be placed, and once it has been, the intramedullary canal of the humerus is identified and subsequently reamed and/or broached according to the protocols for the implant. Trial components are placed and stability and motion should be verified prior to placement of the final components.

4.6. Closure

Once the components have been placed, the shoulder should be reduced and taken through a full range of motion to ensure adequate stability and range of motion. The wound should be irrigated copiously with normal saline and any topical antibiotics should be placed in the wound. If a drain is desired, it should be placed prior to wound closure. The most important aspect of wound closure is the repair of the deltoid muscle back to the acromion. The method for repair of the deltoid back to the acromion will vary slightly based on the method that the deltoid was detached from the acromion.

If the deltoid was peeled subperiosteally off the acromion, it must be repaired using a large-diameter, non-absorbable suture in a transosseous fashion. Many large-diameter suture needles are strong enough to pass through the acromion without using a power drill; however, if the bone is hard, a drill may be used [44]. The suture should be passed through the deltoid with sufficient purchase to ensure that the suture does not pull through the muscle. If the acromial osteotomy was utilized, suture should be passed around the fleck of the acromion with sufficient purchase in the deltoid to again prevent pulling through the suture within the substance of the deltoid.

Once the deltoid has been adequately repaired to the acromion, the deltoid raphe should be sutured with a 0 vicryl or polydioxanone (PDS) suture in a running whipstitch or figure-of-eight interupted fashion. Care should again be taken to avoid suturing below the previously placed stay suture to avoid damaging the axillary nerve. With the raphe closed, the subcutaneous layer may be closed with an absorbable 2-0 suture and the skin with a nylon, running monocryl or other method of skin closure. A dry dressing or an incisional vacuum should be placed over the wound and the arm placed into a sling with abduction pillow prior to awakening the patient.

4.7. Advantages

The anterosuperior approach provides several advantages to the deltopectoral approach. Perhaps, the greatest of these is the subscapularis sparing nature of the approach. Though originally Mackenzie described the approach with a subscapularis tenotomy, modern-day surgeons have typically modified this approach to spare the subscapularis. Utilizing a subscapularis tenotomy with adequate repair, Miller et al. showed, both clinically and functionally, that the subscapularis was deficient following shoulder arthroplasty in a majority of cases [45]. Jackson et al. showed high re-rupture rates following repair of a tenotomy using ultrasound and then showed that it was associated with decreased function [46]. Furthermore, early literature has shown that subscapularis-deficient shoulders have higher rates of instability [36], though other studies have shown no significant difference [47].

The anterosuperior lateral approach is also superior in terms of exposure to the posterior structures of the shoulder, including the posterior glenoid and the rotator cuff. This exposure may be particularly useful for three- or four-part proximal humerus fractures where the greater tuberosity fragment attached to the rotator cuff is pulled posterior and superior [44]. The exposure of the glenoid via the anterosuperior approach is, historically, felt to be superior to that of the deltopectoral approach. It allows for visualization of the entire glenoid and for better sagittal positioning of the glenoid component. Furthermore, it allows for easier preparation of the glenoid, particularly in obese patients and in cases where the glenoid may be retroverted.

4.8. Disadvantages

Despite having superior exposure of the glenoid as a whole, exposure of the inferior aspect of the glenoid is more difficult via the anterosuperior approach. As such, it is more difficult to provide sufficient inferior tilt of the glenoid component which may lead to scapular notching and subsequent failure of the glenoid component [35, 48, 49]. Furthermore, the presence of inferior osteophytes is a relative contraindication to this approach due to the extreme difficulty in accessing and removing these osteophytes. In addition, there is a theoretical disadvantage of weakening of the deltoid through this exposure. There is no literature regarding the status of the deltoid repair or deltoid function after using this approach. However, because the repair of the deltoid to the acromion relies on muscle-to-bone healing, the deltoid may have difficulty healing and subsequent dysfunction. This could be particularly problematic when placing a reverse shoulder prosthesis that relies on intact deltoid function to be successful. If a fleck of acromion is taken, there is a theoretical risk of iatrogenic fracture to the acromion when harvesting the fleck. However, one study, comparing the two approaches, found a significantly higher rate of acromion fracture with the deltopectoral approach compared to the anterosuperior approach [7]. A final disadvantage of the anterosuperior approach is the inability to extend the incision distal if a periprosthetic humeral fracture is encountered. Because it does not utilize an intermuscular plane, it is not able to be extended to the midshaft of the humerus. Furthermore, at the distal aspect of the incision lies the axillary nerve. Webb, in his surgical technique for proximal humerus fractures, states that should distal exposure be needed, the axillary nerve can be identified, protected, and a plate may be placed underneath the axillary nerve [44].

5. Alternate approaches

The deltopectoral and anterosuperior approaches are by and large the most commonly used approaches for shoulder arthroplasty; however, there are other approaches to the glenohumeral joint which have been described in the literature. Lafosse et al. described an approach for anatomic total shoulder arthroplasty that spares all of the rotator-cuff tendons and is performed through the rotator interval [50]. The approach mimics that of the anterosuperior approach in that the deltoid is split in line with its fibers in the raphe between the anterior and middle portions of the deltoids. Again, similar to the anterosuperior approach, the authors had difficulty removing the inferior osteophytes as well as performing an anatomic humeral neck cut and sizing of the humeral head. Two-year follow-up data from this approach do show promising results, though no comparison was made to the deltopectoral approach.

Bellamy et al. performed a cadaveric study analyzing more minimally invasive approaches to the subscapularis including a partial tenotomy and a subscapularis split [51]. In this study, they measured the average area of the glenoid and the humerus that they could visualize through each of these approaches. They found that all of these approaches had adequate exposure of the glenoid; however, the split provided poor exposure of the humerus for humeral-based procedures, while the partial tenotomy provided sufficient exposure.

Gagey et al. presented the results of 53 patients who underwent anatomic total shoulder arthroplasty over a 6-year span via a posterolateral approach [52]. This approach begins with the patient in the lateral decubitus position and a posterior incision is made and carried down between the raphe of the posterior and middle portions of the deltoid. The bursa is then released to identify the tendons of the external rotators. The tendons are then removed via an osteotomy of the greater tuberosity. This allows for exposure to the glenohumeral joint. The osteotomy is then repaired in a manner similar to the lesser tuberosity osteotomy described in the deltopectoral section. Adequate exposure was achieved for placement of shoulder arthroplasty components; however, the authors did note two cases of posterior deltoid atrophy that was unexplained. Brodsky described a modified approach that utilizes the internervous interval between the infraspinatus and the teres minor which allows for preservation of the external rotators [53]. However, no literature exists, which shows that this interval would be feasible for use with shoulder arthroplasty.

A cadaveric study in England compared these three alternative approaches and they found that the posterior approach to the glenohumeral joint provided significantly improved exposure compared to a subscapularis-splitting approach or an approach through the rotator interval [54]. They also measured the average force of retraction on the rotator cuff utilizing these approaches and found that significantly more force was placed on the rotator cuff by retractors in the subscapularis-splitting approach. Before any of these approaches will supplant the deltopectoral or anterosuperior approaches, more research needs to be performed to ensure that good outcomes with minimal morbidity can be achieved through these approaches.

6. Conclusion

While the deltopectoral approach is more widely used than the anterosuperior approach, particularly in shoulder arthroplasty, copious literature exists regarding the outcomes and complications for both of these approaches. Both approaches have been shown to be successful in their utilization for shoulder arthroplasty [1, 7, 55, 56]. The deltopectoral approach has been associated with an increased risk of instability, particularly when the subscapularis is deficient. The anterosuperior approach has been shown to have higher rates of scapular notching. Each approach has its own distinct advantages and disadvantages; however, each can be used successfully in the setting of shoulder arthroplasty. Surgeon preference and comfort with the approach should be the most important deciding factor when choosing an approach.

Author details

Brian W. Sager and Michael Khazzam*

*Address all correspondence to: drkhazzam@yahoo.com

University of Texas Southwestern Medical Center, Department of Orthopaedic Surgery, Dallas, Texas, USA

References

[1] Bufquin T, Hersan A, Hubert L, Massin P. Reverse shoulder arthroplasty for the treatment of three- and four-part fractures of the proximal humerus in the elderly: A prospective review of 43 cases with a short-term follow-up. The Journal of Bone and Joint Surgery British. 2007;89(4):516-520

[2] Cuff D, Pupello D, Virani N, Levy J, Frankle M. Reverse shoulder arthroplasty for the treatment of rotator cuff deficiency. The Journal of Bone and Joint Surgery America. 2008;**90**(6):1244-1251

[3] Green A, Norris TR. Shoulder arthroplasty for advanced glenohumeral arthritis after anterior instability repair. Journal of Shoulder and Elbow Surgery. 2001;**10**(6):539-545

[4] Mulieri P, Dunning P, Klein S, Pupello D, Frankle M. Reverse shoulder arthroplasty for the treatment of irreparable rotator cuff tear without glenohumeral arthritis. The Journal of Bone and Joint Surgery America. 2010;**92**(15):2544-2556

[5] Neer CS, 2nd. Replacement arthroplasty for glenohumeral osteoarthritis. The Journal of Bone and Joint Surgery America. 1974;**56**(1):1-13

[6] Carayon A, Cornet L, Huet R. Deltopectoral approach: Value and indications in vasculo-nervous lesions of the axilla. Medecine Tropicale (Mars). 1958;**18**(4):708-719

[7] Mole D, Wein F, Dezaly C, Valenti P, Sirveaux F. Surgical technique: The anterosuperior approach for reverse shoulder arthroplasty. Clinical Orthopaedics and Related Research. 2011;**469**(9):2461-2468

[8] Li X, Eichinger JK, Hartshorn T, Zhou H, Matzkin EG, Warner JP. A comparison of the lateral decubitus and beach-chair positions for shoulder surgery: Advantages and complications. Journal of the American Academy of Orthopaedic Surgeons. 2015;**23**(1):18-28

[9] Hynson JM, Tung A, Guevara JE, Katz JA, Glick JM, Shapiro WA. Complete airway obstruction during arthroscopic shoulder surgery. Anesthesia & Analgesia. 1993;**76**(4): 875-878

[10] Pohl A, Cullen DJ. Cerebral ischemia during shoulder surgery in the upright position: A case series. Journal of Clinical Anesthesiology. 2005;**17**(6):463-469

[11] Yano K, Minoda Y, Sakawa A, Kuwano Y, Kondo K, Fukushima W, Tada K. Positive nasal culture of methicillin-resistant Staphylococcus aureus (MRSA) is a risk factor for surgical site infection in orthopedics. Acta Orthopaedica. 2009;**80**(4):486-490

[12] Bosco JA, Bookman J, Slover J, Edusei E, Levine B. Principles of antibiotic prophylaxis in total joint arthroplasty: Current concepts. Journal of the American Academy of Orthopaedic Surgeons. 2015;**23**(8):e27-35

[13] Friedman RJ, Gordon E, Butler RB, Mock L, Dumas B. Tranexamic acid decreases blood loss after total shoulder arthroplasty. Journal of Shoulder and Elbow Surgery. 2016;**25**(4):614-618

[14] Gillespie R, Shishani Y, Joseph S, Streit JJ, Gobezie R. Neer Award 2015: A randomized, prospective evaluation on the effectiveness of tranexamic acid in reducing blood loss after total shoulder arthroplasty. Journal of Shoulder and Elbow Surgery. 2015;**24**(11):1679-1684

[15] Sanchez-Sotelo J, Sperling JW, Rowland CM, Cofield RH. Instability after shoulder arthroplasty: Results of surgical treatment. The Journal of Bone and Joint Surgery America. 2003;**85-A**(4):622-631

[16] Buecking B, Mohr J, Bockmann B, Zettl R, Ruchholtz S. Deltoid-split or deltopectoral approaches for the treatment of displaced proximal humeral fractures? Clinical Orthopaedics and Related Research. 2014;**472**(5):1576-1585

[17] Gerber C, Pennington SD, Yian EH, Pfirrmann CA, Werner CM, Zumstein MA. Lesser tuberosity osteotomy for total shoulder arthroplasty. Surgical technique. The Journal of Bone and Joint Surgery America. 2006;**88**(Suppl 1 Pt 2):170-177

[18] Habermeyer P, Magosch P, Lichtenberg S. Recentering the humeral head for glenoid deficiency in total shoulder arthroplasty. Clinical Orthopaedics and Related Research. 2007;**457**:124-132

[19] Harryman DT, 2nd. Common surgical approaches to the shoulder. Instructional Course Lectures. 1992;**41**:3-11

[20] Radkowski CA, Richards RS, Pietrobon R, Moorman CT, 3rd. An anatomic study of the cephalic vein in the deltopectoral shoulder approach. Clinical Orthopaedics and Related Research. 2006;**442**:139-142

[21] Boardman ND, 3rd, Cofield RH. Neurologic complications of shoulder surgery. Clinical Orthopaedics and Related Research. 1999;**368**:44-53

[22] Gerber C, Yian EH, Pfirrmann CA, Zumstein MA, Werner CM. Subscapularis muscle function and structure after total shoulder replacement with lesser tuberosity osteotomy and repair. The Journal of Bone and Joint Surgery America. 2005;**87**(8):1739-1745

[23] Torchia ME, Cofield RH, Settergren CR. Total shoulder arthroplasty with the Neer prosthesis: Long-term results. Journal of Shoulder and Elbow Surgery. 1997;**6**(6):495-505

[24] Armstrong A, Lashgari C, Teefey S, Menendez J, Yamaguchi K, Galatz LM. Ultrasound evaluation and clinical correlation of subscapularis repair after total shoulder arthroplasty. Journal of Shoulder and Elbow Surgery. 2006;**15**(5):541-548

[25] Scalise JJ, Ciccone J, Iannotti JP. Clinical, radiographic, and ultrasonographic comparison of subscapularis tenotomy and lesser tuberosity osteotomy for total shoulder arthroplasty. The Journal of Bone and Joint Surgery America. 2010;**92**(7):1627-1634

[26] Defranco MJ, Higgins LD, Warner JJ. Subscapularis management in open shoulder surgery. Journal of the American Academy of Orthopaedic Surgeons. 2010;**18**(12):707-717

[27] Lapner PL, Sabri E, Rakhra K, Bell K, Athwal GS. Healing rates and subscapularis fatty infiltration after lesser tuberosity osteotomy versus subscapularis peel for exposure during shoulder arthroplasty. Journal of Shoulder and Elbow Surgery. 2013;**22**(3):396-402

[28] Giuseffi SA, Wongtriratanachai P, Omae H, Cil A, Zobitz ME, An KN, Sperling JW, Steinmann SP. Biomechanical comparison of lesser tuberosity osteotomy versus subscapularis tenotomy in total shoulder arthroplasty. Journal of Shoulder and Elbow Surgery. 2012;**21**(8):1087-1095

[29] Van den Berghe GR, Nguyen B, Patil S, D'Lima DD, Mahar A, Pedowitz R, Hoenecke HR. A biomechanical evaluation of three surgical techniques for subscapularis repair. Journal of Shoulder and Elbow Surgery. 2008;**17**(1):156-161

[30] Van Thiel GS, Wang VM, Wang FC, Nho SJ, Piasecki DP, Bach BR, Jr., Romeo AA. Biomechanical similarities among subscapularis repairs after shoulder arthroplasty. Journal of Shoulder and Elbow Surgery. 2010;**19**(5):657-663

[31] Iannotti JP, Gabriel JP, Schneck SL, Evans BG, Misra S. The normal glenohumeral relationships. An anatomical study of one hundred and forty shoulders. The Journal of Bone and Joint Surgery America. 1992;**74**(4):491-500

[32] Duparc F, Bocquet G, Simonet J, Freger P. Anatomical basis of the variable aspects of injuries of the axillary nerve (excluding the terminal branches in the deltoid muscle). Surgical and Radiologic Anatomy. 1997;**19**(3):127-132

[33] Loomer R, Graham B. Anatomy of the axillary nerve and its relation to inferior capsular shift. Clinical Orthopaedics and Related Research. 1989;**243**:100-105

[34] Kelly JD, 2nd, Humphrey CS, Norris TR. Optimizing glenosphere position and fixation in reverse shoulder arthroplasty, Part One: The twelve-mm rule. Journal of Shoulder and Elbow Surgery. 2008;**17**(4):589-594

[35] Gillespie RJ, Garrigues GE, Chang ES, Namdari S, Williams GR, Jr. Surgical exposure for reverse total shoulder arthroplasty: Differences in approaches and outcomes. Orthopedic Clinics of North America. 2015;**46**(1):49-56

[36] Edwards TB, Williams MD, Labriola JE, Elkousy HA, Gartsman GM, O'Connor DP. Subscapularis insufficiency and the risk of shoulder dislocation after reverse shoulder arthroplasty. Journal of Shoulder and Elbow Surgery. 2009;**18**(6):892-896

[37] Trappey GJT, O'Connor DP, Edwards TB. What are the instability and infection rates after reverse shoulder arthroplasty? Clinical Orthopaedics and Related Research. 2011;**469**(9):2505-2511

[38] Miller BS, Joseph TA, Noonan TJ, Horan MP, Hawkins RJ. Rupture of the subscapularis tendon after shoulder arthroplasty: Diagnosis, treatment, and outcome. Journal of Shoulder and Elbow Surgery. 2005;**14**(5):492-496

[39] Lynch NM, Cofield RH, Silbert PL, Hermann RC. Neurologic complications after total shoulder arthroplasty. Journal of Shoulder and Elbow Surgery. 1996;**5**(1):53-61

[40] Mackenzie D. The antero-superior exposure for total shoulder replacement. Orthopaedics and Traumatology. 1993;**2**(2):71-77

[41] Warner JP, Krushell RJ, Masquelet A, Gerber C. Anatomy and relationships of the suprascapular nerve: Anatomical constraints to mobilization of the supraspinatus and infraspinatus muscles in the management of massive rotator-cuff tears. The Journal of Bone and Joint Surgery America. 1992;**74**(1):36-45

[42] Burkhead WZ, Jr, Scheinberg RR, Box G. Surgical anatomy of the axillary nerve. Journal of Shoulder and Elbow Surgery. 1992;**1**(1):31-36

[43] Neer CS, 2nd. Anterior acromioplasty for the chronic impingement syndrome in the shoulder: A preliminary report. The Journal of Bone and Joint Surgery America. 1972;**54**(1):41-50

[44] Webb MF, Funk L. An anterosuperior approach for proximal humerus fractures. Techniques in Shoulder & Elbow Surgery. 2006;**7**(2):77-81

[45] Miller SL, Hazrati Y, Klepps S, Chiang A, Flatow EL. Loss of subscapularis function after total shoulder replacement: A seldom recognized problem. Journal of Shoulder and Elbow Surgery. 2003;**12**(1):29-34

[46] Jackson JD, Cil A, Smith J, Steinmann SP. Integrity and function of the subscapularis after total shoulder arthroplasty. Journal of Shoulder and Elbow Surgery. 2010;**19**(7):1085-1090

[47] Clark JC, Ritchie J, Song FS, Kissenberth MJ, Tolan SJ, Hart ND, Hawkins RJ. Complication rates, dislocation, pain, and postoperative range of motion after reverse shoulder arthroplasty in patients with and without repair of the subscapularis. Journal of Shoulder and Elbow Surgery. 2012;**21**(1):36-41

[48] Levigne C, Boileau P, Favard L, Garaud P, Mole D, Sirveaux F, Walch G. Scapular notching in reverse shoulder arthroplasty. Journal of Shoulder and Elbow Surgery. 2008;**17**(6):925-935

[49] Melis B, DeFranco M, Ladermann A, Mole D, Favard L, Nerot C, Maynou C, Walch G. An evaluation of the radiological changes around the Grammont reverse geometry shoulder arthroplasty after eight to 12 years. The Journal of Bone and Joint Surgery British. 2011;**93**(9):1240-1246

[50] Lafosse L, Schnaser E, Haag M, Gobezie R. Primary total shoulder arthroplasty performed entirely thru the rotator interval: Technique and minimum two-year outcomes. Journal of Shoulder and Elbow Surgery. 2009;**18**(6):864-873

[51] Bellamy JL, Johnson AE, Beltran MJ, Hsu JR, Skeletal Trauma Research Consortium (STReC). Quantification of the exposure of the glenohumeral joint from the minimally invasive to more invasive subscapularis approach to the anterior shoulder: A cadaveric study. Journal of Shoulder and Elbow Surgery. 2014;**23**(6):895-901

[52] Gagey O, Spraul JM, Vinh TS. Posterolateral approach of the shoulder: Assessment of 50 cases. Journal of Shoulder and Elbow Surgery. 2001;**10**(1):47-51

[53] Brodsky JW, Tullos HS, Gartsman GM. Simplified posterior approach to the shoulder joint. A technical note. The Journal of Bone and Joint Surgery America. 1987;**69**(5):773-774

[54] Amirthanayagam TD, Amis AA, Reilly P, Emery RJ. Rotator cuff-sparing approaches for glenohumeral joint access: An anatomic feasibility study. Journal of Shoulder and Elbow Surgery. 2017;**26**(3):512-520

[55] Levy O, Copeland SA. Cementless surface replacement arthroplasty of the shoulder. 5- to 10-year results with the Copeland mark-2 prosthesis. The Journal of Bone and Joint Surgery British. 2001;**83**(2):213-221

[56] Matsen FA, 3rd, Boileau P, Walch G, Gerber C, Bicknell RT. The reverse total shoulder arthroplasty. The Journal of Bone and Joint Surgery America. 2007;**89**(3):660-667

Permissions

List of Contributors

Alexander Golant, Tony Quach, Kevin Jiang and Jeffrey E. Rosen
Department of Orthopedics and Rehabilitation, NewYork-Presbyterian Queens, New York City, USA

Daiji Kano
Department of Surgery, NewYork-Presbyterian Queens, New York City, USA

Raoul Saggini
Department of Medical Oral and Biotechnological Sciences, School of Specialty in Physical and Rehabilitation Medicine, "Gabriele d'Annunzio" University, Chieti, Italy

Simona Maria Carmignano, Lucia Cosenza and Tommaso Palermo
School of Specialty in Physical and Rehabilitation Medicine, "Gabriele d'Annunzio" University, Chieti, Italy

Rosa Grazia Bellomo
Physical and Rehabilitation Medicine, Department of Medical Oral and Biotechnological Sciences, "Gabriele d'Annunzio" University, Chieti, Italy

José Miguel Esparza Miñana
Escuela de Doctorado, Universidad Católica de Valencia San Vicente Mártir, Hospital de Manises, Valencia, Spain

Roger Hackney
Spire Hospital, Leeds, United Kingdom

Piotr Lesniewski and Paul Cowling
Chapel Allerton Hospital LTH, Leeds, United Kingdom

Taiceer A. Abdulwahab
Department of Orthopaedic Surgery, Mediclinic City Hospital, Dubai, United Arab Emirates

William D. Murrell and Frank Z. Jenio
Sapphire Surgery and Medical Centre, Emirates Hospitals Group, Dubai, United Arab Emirates

Navneet Bhangra
Mediclinic Mirdif, Dubai, United Arab Emirates

Gerard A. Malanga and Michael Stafford
Rutgers School of Medicine – New Jersey Medical School, New Jersey, USA

Nitin B. Jain
Vanderbilt University School of Medicine, Nashville, USA

Olivier Verborgt
AZ Monica Hospital, Antwerp, Belgium

Sydney C. Cryder
Department of Medicine, Ohio University, Heritage College of Osteopathic Medicine, Athens, United States

Samuel E. Perry
Department of Graduate Medical Education, Adena Health System, Chillicothe, United States

Elizabeth A. Beverly
Department of Family Medicine, Ohio University, Heritage College of Osteopathic Medicine, Athens, United States

Omkar P. Kulkarni and Satish B. Sonar
Dr. PDM Medical College, Amravati, India

Brian W. Sager and Michael Khazzam
University of Texas Southwestern Medical Center, Department of Orthopaedic Surgery, Dallas, Texas, USA

Index

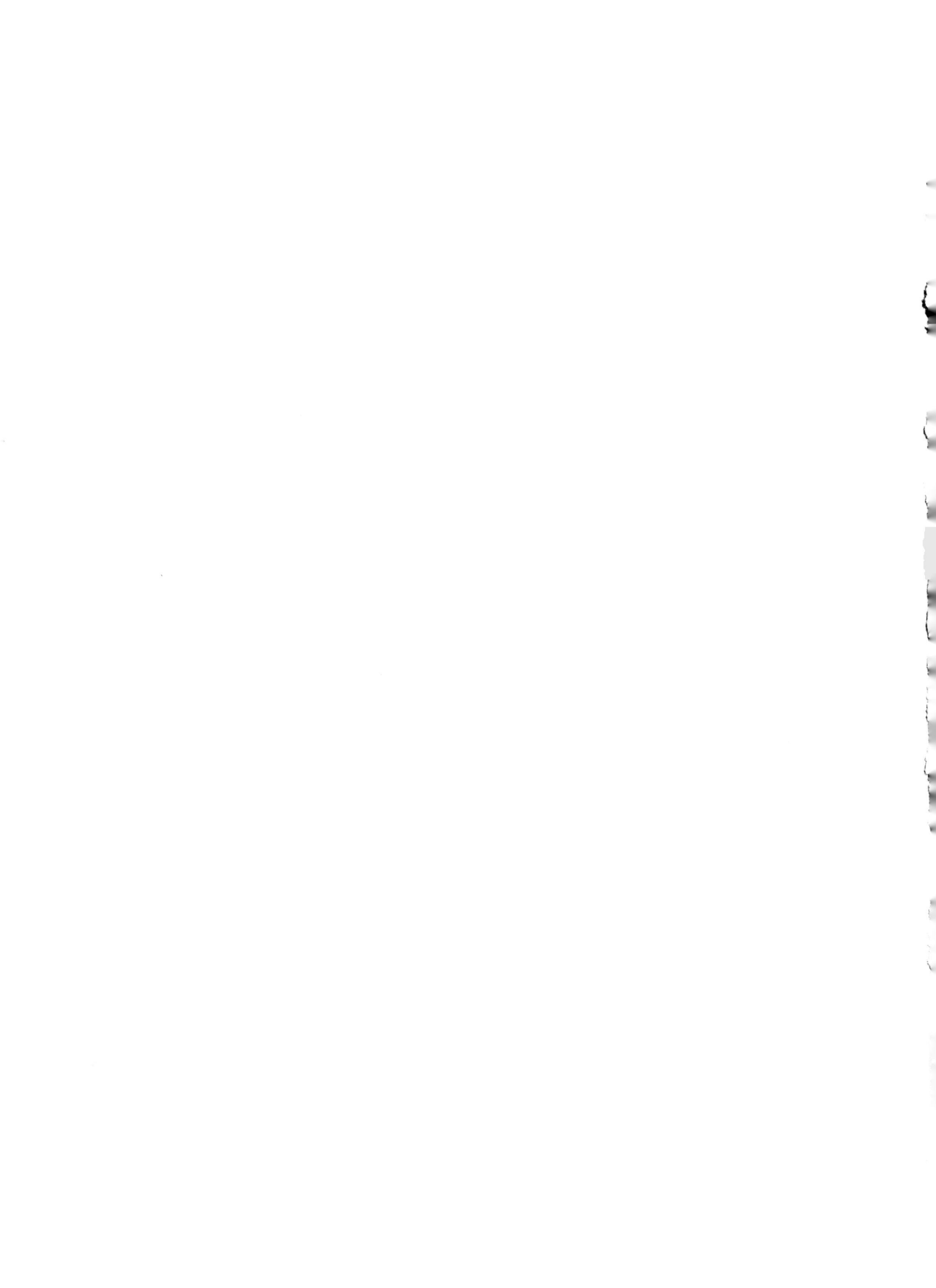